What's Wrong with My Child?

ENDORSEMENTS

Any mother with children with medical needs will be able to identify with Elizabeth's struggle to find answers and to help her children get well. You will recognize in her the traits of a fellow warrior mom.

The issue Elizabeth addresses is of grave importance not only for parents of special-needs kids, but for anyone dealing with health challenges.

It is my opinion that children with Down syndrome are disproportionately afflicted by the bacteria Elizabeth highlights in this book, with only a tiny fraction of the parents being aware of the situation. This may be the root of severe behavior problems, obsessive-compulsive disorder, and why your child might not be talking.

Scary as it may sound, there are answers. Elizabeth has spent countless hours ferreting out the facts for us. I applaud her for her perseverance and unwavering focus which has helped other families not having to go through all she did when looking for answers

Please spread the word so other families can benefit, too. We are in this together!

Andi Durkin
President: Down Syndrome OPTIONs
Blogger at Down Syndrome: A Day-to-Day Guide

Elizabeth's message unveils how the corruption of a very few may have global consequences. The connections she makes go far beyond PANS/PANDAS and is a clarion call to physicians and parents alike not to settle for easy answers. Far too many families are facing mysteries such as this and it is time to look at the root.

Judy A. Mikovits, PhD
Research Scientist
Author, *Plague of Corruption*, *Plague*, and
The Case against the Masks

I believe that the problem Elizabeth identified played a role in my son Erik's battle with mental illness that led to addiction, trauma, and ultimately death. I knew there was something wrong, but no one could get to the underlying cause. The opportunity to know what was wrong with my son was stolen from me.

I pray this book will help families and give hope to the young Eriks of the future. Not one other person needs to go down the same tragic path.

Cindy Blom
Grief and Addiction Coach

Since 2007, I've been involved with the treatment of substance abuse. I've seen thousands of addicts attempt recovery. It never made sense to me why some couldn't get better no matter how hard they tried. Once I read Elizabeth's book, I immediately put the pieces together [making a connection between being infected and being addicted.]

This information needs to available to all who may be affected. Everyone needs the knowledge to have the power to take charge of your health.

Tina Cartwright
Co-Founder, American Addiction Centers

Several years ago, I listened to Elizabeth talking about her son, Cody. Not long after that, I learned about a friend's son who was struggling with severe behavioral issues. He had been sent to a military school. It sounded exactly like what Cody had gone through, so I raised the question of PANDAS to my friend. They were skeptical, so I sent them Elizabeth's [earlier] book. Recently, I learned that they pursued the possibility and are now treating him medically for PANS/PANDAS, and he is getting better!

I trust that this book will likewise help many families so their children can be healed.

Lisa McIntyre, Brentwood, TN

As a client, I observed Elizabeth's struggles for years. Her battles with the medical system, insurance, and then the courts were more than most could bare. Yet she was relentless, and in the end, she uncovered the truth. This book is a must-read for anyone who is battling to get to the root of family disease.

Brenda Weiss
Cardiac Nurse

As a client at Elizabeth's medi-spa, I had the honor of getting regular updates on Elizabeth's battle trying to identify the root behind her son's unusual health challenges. Elizabeth was tenacious in pursuing an understanding of her son's symptoms, the origin of these symptoms, and finding someone who would work with her to develop a treatment plan.

Unfortunately, there were many who were not sympathetic regarding her quest. She was written off as being eccentric, obsessive, and as crazy as her son. Still, against formidable odds, she remained tireless in defending her family against mental health professionals and the justice system. After a journey of several years, her son is now doing very well. Elizabeth's fight for Cody has been an example for us all.

Elizabeth not only has an insatiable desire not only to learn she also wants to help others who can benefit from what she had learned.

Rebeccah Land, PhD
Clinical Social Worker, Licensed Clinical Social Worker

The ever-increasing list of diagnoses my son kept getting didn't sit right with me. How could one child have ADHD, ODD, OCD, enuresis, sleep apnea, periodic limb movement disorder, academic decline, and more? As the diagnoses piled up, so did the medicines to treat them.

There had to be a connection between the various issues, but no doctor was able to find it. Ultimately, I was the one who identified

PANS/PANDAS in my son. He had all the classic symptoms. My pediatrician was hesitant to affirm my suspicions at first but agreed to let me go through the diagnostic process.

Among many other interventions, we started chiropractic treatment and neurofeedback, and the neurofeedback practitioner suggested that I meet with Elizabeth. Within just six weeks of being treated by Elizabeth, my son was no longer using a CPAP, his restless leg syndrome was gone, and the psych meds we relied on so heavily were no longer needed. Over the following months, he became successful in school, both academically and behaviorally. He made several friends and was finally able to spend a night away from home. Now, we can even take family trips!

Though I saw it with my own eyes, I am still in disbelief.

Athena West
Publisher and Owner of a Luxury Magazine

My healthy sixteen-year-old son contracted mycoplasma pneumonia. A few months later, he was diagnosed with schizophrenia. It seemed obvious that the issues were connected; I just didn't know how. And I wasn't willing to simply accept a lifelong diagnosis if there were a solution.

Five years later, I came across Elizabeth's [first] book. A glimmer of hope was sparked, and I reached out to her. Elizabeth agreed to help. Turns out that my son did not have schizophrenia; he had PANS/PANDAS.

It's been a long road, but my son no longer hears voices. Thank you, Elizabeth, for giving me my son back.

Shannon Longstead
PANS/PANDAS Mom

My husband was a major in the United States Air Force Reserves. He served as a flight surgeon at Selfridge Air Force Base, Michigan, where he took care of active-duty members who were returning from the First Gulf War. Since that time, my husband, our five children, and I have struggled with immune issues and with strep. Getting all seven of us well became my primary focus.

Elizabeth's findings have helped us tremendously. God speed Elizabeth. Thank you for your tireless efforts in helping us heal.

Suzanne Hollerbach Nelson
Physical Therapist, DM

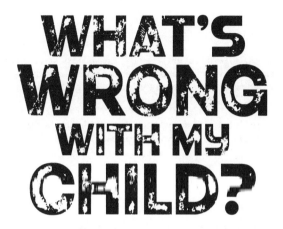

WHAT'S WRONG WITH MY CHILD?

ONE MOTHER'S DESPERATE QUEST
to Uncover What Was Really Wrong with Her Family...
and THE DISTURBING FACTS *She Revealed that Could*
HELP SAVE YOURS

ELIZABETH HARRIS

NEW YORK

LONDON • NASHVILLE • MELBOURNE • VANCOUVER

What's Wrong with My Child?

One Mother's Desperate Quest to Uncover What Was Really Wrong with Her Family ... and The Disturbing Facts She Revealed that Could Help Save Yours

Published in New York, New York, by Morgan James Publishing. Morgan James is a trademark of Morgan James, LLC. www.MorganJamesPublishing.com

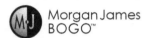

Morgan James BOGO™

A **FREE** ebook edition is available for you or a friend with the purchase of this print book.

CLEARLY SIGN YOUR NAME ABOVE

Instructions to claim your free ebook edition:
1. Visit MorganJamesBOGO.com
2. Sign your name CLEARLY in the space above
3. Complete the form and submit a photo of this entire page
4. You or your friend can download the ebook to your preferred device

ISBN 9781631954979 paperback
ISBN 9781631954986 eBook
Library of Congress Control Number:
2021930808

Cover Design by:
Christopher Kirk
www.GFSstudio.com

Interior Design by:
Chris Treccani
www.3dogcreative.net

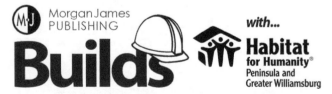

Morgan James is a proud partner of Habitat for Humanity Peninsula and Greater Williamsburg. Partners in building since 2006.

Get involved today! Visit
MorganJamesPublishing.com/giving-back

To my children
I love you all with everything that I am

TABLE OF CONTENTS

Foreword   *xvii*

2003   *xxi*

Chapter 1   A Christmas Jigsaw Puzzle   1

Chapter 2   More Mysteries   15

Chapter 3   Trying to Get Help   25

Chapter 4   Flares   33

Chapter 5   Imperfect Parenting   39

Chapter 6   Patient Dismissal   55

Chapter 7   Up and Down   61

Chapter 8   Little Boxes   71

Chapter 9   Solitary Confinement   85

Chapter 10   Could This Mean Something?   99

Chapter 11   Misdirected Immune Response   109

Chapter 12   A Team of One   119

Chapter 13   Superbug   123

Chapter 14   Genetic Testing   127

Chapter 15   A Broken Immune System   137

Chapter 16   Collecting Data   141

Chapter 17   Contagious—or Not?   147

Chapter 18   Side Effects   151

Chapter 19   Yellow Butterfly   155

Chapter 20   Seeing the Bigger Picture   161

Chapter 21   Connecting the Pieces of the Puzzle   171

Chapter 22   A Simple Test   179
Chapter 23   The Cost of Getting Well   189
Chapter 24   Not Yet Quite to the Finish Line   195
Chapter 25   Helping Others   205

Update   213
Acknowledgments   217
About Elizabeth Harris   223

FOREWORD

first met Elizabeth Harris at a PANDAS conference in Atlanta. She was desperate for answers—like many parents of children with pediatric acute-onset neuropsychiatric disorders associated with streptococcus (PANDAS) are. After a long discussion about her son's case, I agreed to evaluate and treat "Cody."

Cody is fortunate to have a mother who trusted her instinct and would not accept what was happening to her beautiful son. She fought for—and found—answers.

I can happily say through treatment and support, Cody is now grown, free of PANDAS, and leading a very productive life.

This is not the case for every child with PANDAS.

One in every 200 children in the United States will develop symptoms of PANDAS. The typical age of onset ranges from four to thirteen; however, at my clinic, I have treated children even younger than four. In the case of the younger patients, they often have a history of hospitalization, including severe infections.

Many of my patients have either autism or genetic disorders. As a result, pediatricians and parents focus on the primary diagnosis, and the PANDAS remains undiagnosed for far too long while the child and their family suffer in silence.

Thankfully, PANDAS is becoming more recognizable. We diagnose it based on a combination of clinical history, clinical findings, and extensive laboratory testing, including genetic testing.

Many changes arise overnight, frequently following an illness, infection, or a medical procedure. Other changes in a child's behavior may develop gradually and may not be noticed at first by the parent or caregiver.

These signs include:

- a sudden change in personality,
- becoming overly sensitive,
- acting up and acting out,
- withdrawing from peers,
- having trouble with schoolwork,
- regression of skills such as handwriting,
- psychiatric symptoms such as obsessive-compulsive disorder and tic disorders,
- eating disorders, and many more.

Not all children with PANDAS develop the same symptoms, however. As a result, many children are misdiagnosed with having psychiatric disorders. However, many of the psychiatric symptoms are a result of a malfunction in the fever response to infections resulting in neuropsychiatric symptoms.

Some of the children who exhibit these symptoms and come to see me do not, in fact, have PANDAS.

After extensive testing, once we have confirmed that a child *does* have PANDAS, we aim to identify the root problem, and then move forward, aiming to do all we can to help the child, and by extension, the family.

Early evaluation and treatment are crucial for recovery, as in a team approach. If both parents, the primary care physician, as well at the school team can be on board with treating a child, we tend to have greater success.

I commend Elizabeth for her courage and strength, and I pray that this book will offer insight to help save many children from a life of suffering.

Rosario R. Trifiletti, MD PhD
Child Neurologist
The PANDAS/PANS Institute

2003

John and Liz Harris had been married for twelve years when Steven, John's younger brother, called. He was fresh out of yet another drug rehab center, looking for a place to stay.

John was a peaceful guy who went with the flow most of the time but when it came to Steven, he was adamant about helping. Liz reluctantly agreed to open their home to Steven once again. After all, helping people, especially family, was the right thing to do.

Liz tried to stay positive. When Steven was in his right mind, he was hilarious, charming, and full of life. She was cautiously hopeful that this rehab had worked. Steven could help with Kelsey's upcoming tenth birthday party. And Cody, the sweet two-year-old, adored his uncle. And maybe Steven could put his talent as a hairstylist to good use in the new spa and salon she was opening.

Steven had merely been in the home for a week when something weird happened. Painful and bizarre-looking knots that looked like spider bites began erupting on everyone's skin. Liz got the biggest one of all just below her right eyebrow. The physical reminder made her particularly self-conscious. They all ended up going to the doctor, but the cause would remain a mystery.

Just as the boils started clearing up, the family was hit by a second round of mysterious symptoms. This time, they had a loss of appetite, headaches, chills, and fevers. They even had difficulty breathing at times.

Whatever it was, it was hitting them all *hard*.

Since birth, Cody had been prone to pneumonia, and whatever had invaded their home, hit him the worst. He could barely move and refused to eat or drink—even the smallest sips of water.

Although Cody was so dehydrated he could no longer produce tears, Dr. Meneely, their pediatrician, was not too worried. "It sounds like the flu," he said in his thick Irish accent. "Just let it run its course."

When Kelsey also got worse, Liz was desperate. She reached out to her dad to come and help out.

He made the two-hour trip to their house and ended up taking Kelsey to the hospital where she was diagnosed with pleurisy, an inflammation of the membranes that surround the lungs. Kelsey was sent home to recover, and Liz was relieved that her dad offered to stay a few days to help.

Liz remembers finally peeling off the T-shirt and sweatpants she had been living in through the nine-day ordeal and stepping into a long, hot shower—grateful it was over and finally feeling alive again.

But a shower was not going to be enough to wash away everything from that experience.

Little did the Harris family know at the time, but this episode was but the start of a battle against disease, trauma, and substance abuse. Their fifteen-year struggle to put the mysterious medical puzzle together, particularly for Cody, would lead them to countless hospitals—even psych wards and detention centers.

It would cost them their marriage, their sanity, and their family home.

Through this battle, Liz came to learn the truth about an "experiment" gone terribly wrong—one where not only the Harris family was affected.

What she found in her research showed how the wellness of an entire nation had been compromised.

A WORD FROM THE AUTHOR

In our quest for answers, my family and I lived through years of torment and frustration. Along the way, I came to know that there were many other families with stories like ours.

Along the way, I ended up chronicling our experiences, recording conversations with doctors, looking for an answer to the question, "What's wrong with my child?!"

If you are a family like ours, you may be able to relate in many ways. And as a parent, you would know that getting an answer to that question is not enough. Ultimately, **it is about discovering a solution to help your child get better.**

My goal was never to solve a medical mystery. But as you will come to learn, as I kept asking questions, I found more answers than what I had aimed for.

My journey to get to the answers was a long one. It took almost ten years. Once I uncovered the disturbing truth, it took several years of trial and error before we were well.

I was alone, afraid, and fighting for our lives with no help from the medical establishment. But quitting was not an option.

What is represented in this book is but a fraction of the doctor visits, school meetings, court appearances, and sleepless nights. Likewise, I spare you the details around the number of people affected. I merely chronicle the key realizations along the way in the hopes that you will not have to go through what we did to find answers.

This quest was grueling and financially devastating. My desire is for you to be spared the time, the hardship, and the cost. In this book, you will read about stories and events that help depict the gravity of our situation. I came to the realization that Cody was not the only one in the family who was sick. He was diagnosed with PANS/PANDAS/AE[1] while the rest of us all had strange symptoms of varying types. **All of it ended up being connected.**

Had I given up; this story would not have ended well. As parents, we hope that advocating for our children is enough. But, when it is not, we fight hard.

Fortunately, I have a formal education in the sciences and a background in health and wellness. I spent countless hours looking at the hard science behind what doctors were saying. I created spreadsheets to look for patterns in numbers because it just came naturally.

You cannot survive twenty years as a business owner without paying very close attention to the numbers. I read research papers, looking up each unfamiliar word one at a time. You do not have to do that, though. I use simplified terms because I know you are exhausted and overwhelmed. **I want to make it as easy for you as I can.**

Also, I am not a doctor. Out of desperation, I learned what had to be done to get my son and the rest of our family better by

---

1   PANS is an acronym for pediatric acute-onset neuropsychiatric syndrome, and PANDAS is the acronym for pediatric autoimmune neuropsychiatric disorders associated with streptococcal infections. PANDAS a subset of PANS. PANDAS is also sometimes referred to as post-streptococcal autoimmune basal ganglia encephalitis or autoimmune encephalitis (AE) in short. In this book, most references will be to PANS/PANDAS, which you will learn more about in the chapters that follow.

implementing what I learned. Fortunately, you will not have to do that. I will try to point you in the right direction.

Please know this: **The events portrayed in this book are real.** I did not write this book as a vendetta to single out any individual, any doctor, or any hospital.

As I said, I wrote this book so others would not have to go through what we did to get our lives back. Conversations represent the heart of what was said. In most (but not all) cases, I use the real names because, for us, it was real life.

HOW TO READ THIS BOOK

If you are a frustrated parent with limited energy, I get it. It may mean that you can only read a few paragraphs at a time. Read at your own speed. There's no rush.

Keep reading, though. And hang in there. *You are not alone*.

The outcomes of this book are real. I found the solution to Cody's mystery and the medical mysteries my family was facing. The treatment was not easy, nor was it instant. But it was the right answer. And as I write this, it has been more than two years that we have all been well. *There is hope.*

You will learn how we got well—and you will have a choice for how your child (or you) can also get well.

My prayer is that your family, too, will get well.

Elizabeth Harris

CHAPTER 1

A Christmas Jigsaw Puzzle

FALL 2010

"Surprise!" Kelsey shouted as she flung open the front door. "We started decorating. We thought it would make Cody feel better."

Liz smiled proudly at her beautiful, brown-eyed daughter. "That was so thoughtful," Liz said as she helped Cody into the house.

It was nice to have Kelsey home from her first semester at college. Michelle and Adam, the two adopted siblings, were sitting at the dining room table sorting ornaments. "Which one of you got the wreath fastened to the front door?" Liz wanted to know. "That's no easy task."

Michelle perked up in her chair, "I did mom! I'm thirteen, you know. I can do stuff like that."

Adam came over to check on Cody, "Are you okay?" Adam had blonde hair and sea blue eyes that reflected his kind and giving spirit. Both boys were eleven, yet Adam was a full foot shorter

1

than Cody. When they were together, nobody would ever guess they were not biological brothers.

"I'm alright," Cody said weakly as Liz helped him onto the couch.

The banister dripped with holiday greenery, and Christmas boxes overflowed with festive trimmings.

"It looks lovely," Liz said. She was beaming as she took in the sight before her, and she was delighted to see Kelsey in the holiday spirit. Their relationship had been rocky for a while, but it was on the mend. Divorce can be hard on everyone, and Kelsey had offloaded the brunt of her anger on her mother.

Recently, though, Kelsey had decided to move back into the guest suite and attend the local community college. Things seemed as if things may be turning around for Liz and the kids.

"What did the doctor say?" Kelsey wanted to know.

Liz sighed. "Dr. Meneely said Cody has strep *again*. He gave him amoxicillin—as usual." She placed a pharmacy bag on the kitchen table. "Your ADHD[2] meds are in there, too," she said to Kelsey, pointing to the bag.

Michelle hung the last stocking. "Did you remember the candy?" she was eager to know.

"I sure did," Liz smiled and tossed her a Godiva chocolate bar. But Adam caught it and ran with Michelle on his heels. "Adam, I got you some Sour Patch Kids," Liz called after them, "but before you guys eat those, I need you to bring me whatever clothes you want to be washed for your dad's tomorrow."

"Okay, Mom!" they called in unison. The kids all had a close relationship with John, and they looked forward to spending time

---

2   Attention deficit hyperactivity disorder (ADHD) is characterized by a lack of attention, excessive activity, and impulsivity inappropriate for the person's age.

with him. John and Liz had been married for nearly nineteen years, but for the last five, John had become increasingly depressed. He did not do much other than lay around watching television. He struggled with work and with Liz's growing anger at his lack of drive.

Although Liz tried counseling to work through her underlying anger, John's unwillingness to contribute became too much. If she were going to raise the kids and pay the bills on her own, she may as well do that without the distraction of constant frustration.

Christmas music drifted through the house as Liz helped Cody get settled on the couch. "You just relax." Liz gently caressed his wavy, sandy brown hair. His Corgi, Rusty, hopped up beside him and got comfortable.

"Mom, my throat really hurts," Cody whispered. Although her son's excruciating stomach pains had subsided, for now, Liz still felt helpless. Nothing seemed to make Cody feel better.

She tucked an afghan snugly around his legs. "Do you want some sherbet?"

Cody just nodded.

Liz handed Cody a bowl and settled nearby with her laptop. She preferred not to work when the kids were out of school, but she had a deadline to meet. The recession of 2008 had taken a toll, and Liz needed a home run to get back on track.

"Mom, I put my clothes in the washer," Michelle announced as she licked a bit of chocolate from her finger. "Can I help Kelsey decorate the tree?"

"For sure… after you wash up!" Liz was glad that Michelle and Adam were helping decorate their home for Christmas. They had been spending a lot of time alone in their rooms lately. The Harris family adopted them two years earlier. Coming from a traumatic foster-home situation, things had not been easy for them, nor was watching Liz and John go through a divorce. But here they were, having fun decorating the home. Maybe the therapy was helping.

Liz was hoping with all her heart that they were feeling safe and stable. She did her best to make sure the kids were transitioning well, that they were healthy—emotionally *and* physically.

MOM, BUSINESS OWNER, INVENTOR

As the owner of La Bella, a successful high-end spa, Liz was considered an expert in the field of cellulite reduction and body contouring. She was eager to hit the international market with her newest invention—an innovative body-contouring device called CelluSleek. The launch was around the corner, and Liz was confident that this would be a game-changer for her business.

Liz had always loved science. She had a biology degree with a chemistry minor and had been on track for medical school. But during her patient-care internship, she helped develop a cardiac rehabilitation program and fell in love with the fitness and spa business where she happily remained ever since.

ENOUGH IS ENOUGH

"Are you done, Cody?" Kelsey asked, wanting to make room on the coffee table for the Christmas boxes. The melted sherbet had barely been touched.

"Yeah… I'm not hungry," Cody whispered.

"If Uncle Steven were here, he'd get you to eat," Kelsey giggled.

Liz flashed Kelsey a sharp look. "Let's not bring him up."

She had kicked Steven out a few months earlier after another of his epic "storms of madness" that seemed to be getting progressively darker and scarier.

The real Steven was indeed great with the kids. With his theatrical ways, he was somehow able to coax Cody into eating—

even during the times where Cody simply was not hungry, which sometimes went on for weeks on end.

Even though Liz needed help with the children, she couldn't risk the dangers of having him there after he fell apart *again*. She knew the kids would miss their uncle as would she. But it was the best decision for everyone, so Liz had to ask him to leave.

FOCUSED AND FIXATED

With a box full of ornaments, Michelle pushed past Cody who was now standing in the middle of the living room. He had zeroed in on his favorite flannel shirt. He carefully unbuttoned it and took it off. Then he slowly slipped it back on.

Cody fixated on the buttons and made sure the red and black plaids lined up perfectly. Then he started over. Unbutton it. Take it off. Put it back on and button it carefully. Over and over.

"What are you doing up?" Liz patted his back reassuringly. "Dr. Meneely said you're supposed to rest. Lie back down, honey."

Cody couldn't seem to relax; he kept getting back up. He stared at his feet as he took evenly spaced steps through the doorway that separated the living room from the breakfast nook. As he stepped from the carpet onto the hardwood floor, he put one foot in front of the other for a few steps before turning around and continuing in the other direction.

Liz looked up from her laptop. "What in the world are you doing?"

"Well, I have to make sure my right foot goes first," he explained as if this were nothing out of the ordinary.

What?

"And I can't step on any of those lines on the floor."

After she watched him complete twenty-three more rounds, Liz called Dr. Meneely's office. "Something's *seriously* wrong with Cody. It's more than a sore throat."

"Well, just let us know if he gets any worse," the nurse responded in a monotone voice.

Any worse?

Liz tried to concentrate on her work but was distracted by Cody's antics. After insisting she boil his toothbrush to kill all the germs and dry his jeans—even though they were not wet—Cody moved on to a new obsession. He dragged the dining room chairs to the middle of the living room, organized them into a perfect rectangle, and covered them in intricate ways with blankets. It looked like a shelter designed either by an architect or an alien.

She watched as he tucked, straightened, and pulled the blankets back and forth over the chairs. Pillows lined the floor of the tent in a perfect row, but each time he tried to lie down, they moved slightly, so he had to get up and readjust them. Cody announced that he would be sleeping in the "tent."

The other kids had finished decorating the tree. Kelsey had gone back out to the suite, while Michelle and Adam were enjoying popcorn and a movie. Oddly, Cody was not the least bit interested in joining them.

NOT GOING ANYWHERE

The next morning, Liz awoke with an annoying numbness in her hands.

Perhaps the hours I put in writing the CelluSleek manual had aggravated my carpal tunnel.

It took almost an hour before she started feeling tingling in her hands. She had read that immobilizing the wrist helped with carpal tunnel, so she put on wrist braces and cooked breakfast.

She peeked into Cody's tent. Rusty wagged his tail in greeting, but Cody remained fast asleep. Not even the smell of bacon and hot cocoa woke him.

By noon, he still had not eaten, nor had he ventured far from his tent. He had not begun to get ready for the weekend at his dad's house, which was something he normally looked forward to. Instead, Cody spent most of the day in the corner behind a chair or rebuilding the tent.

"You have to see this," Liz insisted when John arrived. "Cody's been messing around in this tent thing all day."

"Cool," John said unfazed. "It's certainly looking Christmassy in here!"

Michelle and Adam clamored down the stairs with their backpacks and pillows. "Dad, have you guys put up your tree? Are there any presents yet?"

John laughed. "You'll have to wait and see. Cody, you got your stuff ready?"

Cody darted from his tent and latched onto Liz's leg. "I'm not going to Dad's!" he insisted.

"Come on, bud," he said. "Kids," he motioned to Michelle and Adam, "go ahead and get in the car."

John reached for Cody's arm, but he stiffened and tightened his grip around Liz's leg.

"What?" John looked at Liz. She shrugged. Cody would not budge. The harder they tried to coax him to let go, the more firmly he held on. Finally, he started to cry.

"Well, I'm not going to force him to come with me," John shrugged. The truth was that his feelings had been hurt. Cody had never acted this way toward him.

"It's okay, he can stay here," Liz said as she stroked Cody's head. "He's just not feeling well today."

HEADING TO THE EMERGENCY ROOM

The next morning, Liz found Rusty pacing the room while Cody was sitting in the corner, eyes wild. "What is wrong, sweetheart?" she asked.

"Bugs are crawling up and down my arms!" He frantically brushed himself with his hands. "It's spiders… It feels like spiders!" His pupils were dilated, and he shook with fear.

When Liz touched his arm, he smacked her hand away.

"There aren't any spiders, honey," she tried assuring him, but she couldn't convince him otherwise.

Am I missing something?

Liz was beside herself with worry. She was watching Cody slowly lose his mind.

How is it that he could be feeling things that weren't there?

She called Dr. Meneely's office for the third time and demanded to speak to him as soon as possible. Within minutes, another doctor called her back.

"I'm Dr. Brooks. How can I help?"

After she launched into the details of the past three days, he said decisively: "This sounds like an acute onset of PANDAS. You need to take him to the emergency room at Vanderbilt Hospital."

Liz was relieved that Dr. Brooks knew what it was. She ran to pack a few things for Cody, and frantically googled "pandas."

Whatever it is, it must be serious.

Other than pages filled with images of giant pandas, she found a website from the National Institute of Mental Health (NIMH) that seemed related. They described it as "pediatric autoimmune neuropsychiatric disorders associated with streptococcal infections."

According to NIMH, PANDAS was a term used to describe children who have obsessive-compulsive disorder (OCD) and/or a tic disorder such as Tourette's syndrome and whose symptoms first appear or worsen following a strep infection.

Several sites explained that such children usually had a dramatic, overnight appearance of symptoms. These could include severe separation anxiety, obsessions and/or compulsions, disordered eating, personality changes, and they become moody and irritable, including having sensory sensitivities. They also have increased urinary frequency, physical or vocal tics, and acute handwriting difficulties.

She looked over at Cody who was still clawing at his arms and whimpering.

Strep throat did this?

Liz called John to explain what was going on. "We are headed to the Vanderbilt emergency room. I'll keep you posted. Can you keep the kids a little longer? Maybe they can stay with you until we know what's going on."

She hugged Cody tightly. "It's okay, son. The doctors will know what to do."

AT THE EMERGENCY ROOM

In the examination room, the staff threw all sorts of odd questions at her. "Has there been any recent trauma?" a nurse asked.

"Well, his father and I just went through a divorce," Liz said and shifted uncomfortably in her chair.

"How did Cody handle it?"

"He was upset, of course. But I don't understand what that has to do with him taking his shirt on and off and hiding in corners thinking there are invisible bugs on him."

"Sometimes trauma can worsen OCD." The woman scribbled in her notebook.

"OCD? What OCD?"

"Has Cody ever arranged things, organized things, or needed to have things a certain way?" the nurse continued.

"Well, I'm a perfectionist," Liz answered, "and Cody is like me. When he was younger, he sometimes spent hours lining up his toy cars. And he's always been picky about his clothes. I don't mean the regular kind of picky. He would cry and get extremely agitated if he felt the least bit uncomfortable. Is that OCD?"

"Yes, those are OCD tendencies. But now it is acute," the nurse explained. "What medications is he taking?"

"Concerta for ADHD and amoxicillin for strep."

As the nurse turned to exit, a tall man entered the room. "I'm the attending physician. I'll be taking care of Cody. I've called neurology for consultation, and they'll be doing some tests."

"We need to see the PANDAS specialist."

"I'll get someone in here."

"Okay," Liz said and sat down next to Cody's bed. She tried to comfort him. Little did she know that the doctor who was being called for was no PANDAS specialist; he was a psychiatrist.

Cody thrashed around on the bed. "Mom, I hate it here. Can you tell them to turn the music off?"

"What music?" Liz gave the doctor a bewildered look.

"He's having auditory hallucinations," the doctor said. "It's when you hear things that aren't there." He wrote on Cody's chart. "We're going to go ahead and admit him."

LOOKING FOR CLUES

Liz listened carefully for clues as to what was going on as nurses, doctors, and students paraded in and out of Cody's room while carrying on their private conversations.

If this puzzle revolved around my son, can I at least see the box, please?

"Ms. Harris, the MRI revealed some slight abnormalities and bilateral maxillary sinus disease," the neurologist told Liz. "We are going to do a spinal tap and draw Cody's blood for anti-streptolysin O and anti-DNase B[3] titer testing."

What are all these tests?! My son had strep, and here he's getting an MRI and a spinal tap and a slew of tests I'd never heard of! How did we get here? How did we get to PANDAS?

After the tests, the chaos finally seemed to subside. Liz snuggled beside Cody as he lay peacefully. After her son drifted off, she pulled out her laptop and jumped back on the NIMH website to research the tests the neurologist had rattled off.

Liz learned that these tests could determine if a strep infection is or has been present. A doctor typically drew the titers—the number of antibodies—from a blood sample when a child was sick and again several weeks later to see if it was rising. If it was, it indicated strong evidence that the recent symptoms were due to strep.

From all the case studies she read, the only common factor she found among people with PANDAS—other than sudden behavioral changes—was the high anti-DNase B titers.

She needed to see Cody's titer numbers.

NO ANSWERS

The spinal tap came back normal, and by day three, the antibiotics they had given Cody intravenously had improved his condition tremendously, though not yet completely.

---

3   Anti-streptolysin O and anti-DNase B are antibodies the immune system produces in response to a strep infection.

"We are going to discharge him today," the doctor announced.

Cody sat up excitedly, but Liz was confused. "Discharge him? We don't have the results of his anti-DNase B titer test yet. How can you discharge him before we know what he has?" She was getting angry.

While the doctor looked at Cody's chart, Liz glanced over his shoulder, seeing the words: *Psychosis resolved.*

"How did you resolve it? No disrespect, sir, but children do not randomly go insane for no reason and then randomly get well. I'd like to know what happened and why."

She turned to her son. "Cody, lie back down."

Fortunately, the results came in while the discharge nurse was completing the paperwork.

"Let's see… Cody's anti-DNase B titers are 1,480," the doctor announced.

"Are you kidding me? That's seven times higher than normal! What do we do? Does he have PANDAS?"

Over time, Liz would learn that since PANDAS had only recently been discussed at the NIMH, not many at Vanderbilt Hospital seemed to be aware of or agree with the fact PANDAS was a legitimate diagnosis.

The nurse came in and launched into the instructions: "Give Cody these antibiotics until they are completely gone. And this should be enough Zoloft to tie you over until you get to see your primary care physician."

Zoloft? Why would they give him an antidepressant for strep?

"Also, for his ADHD meds," the nurse continued, "we're changing his Concerta to Strattera because it's a non-stimulant. It should help to calm him some. He may be a little sore from the spinal tap. If so, give him some ibuprofen." She handed Liz a prescription. "Please follow up with your primary care physician."

Without answers to any of Liz's questions, Cody was sent home.

UNDER ATTACK FROM WITHIN

The ibuprofen did not help to ease the pain from the spinal tap. Hours after Cody was settled in bed, he was still crying. He refused to let his mom as much as touch him.

The wheels in Liz's mind were turning. She remembered learning in college that the strep bacteria were "masters of disguise," that they could morph to appear to be a heart cell, for example—a process called molecular mimicry.

Typically, when the body would detect something foreign, it would create antibodies to attack it. But because of the way the strep mimics the healthy cells, the body would attack the healthy cells along with the strep cells in disguise. The body would launch a full-on autoimmune attack.

Is this what's happening? How does one cell mimic another, anyway? There seems to be much more to how Cody's body is turning on itself.

The first step in working on a jigsaw puzzle is to turn the pieces right side up. You don't sort them or connect them yet. You simply flip the pieces over.

Liz was determined to do that, one piece at a time.

CHAPTER 2

More Mysteries

THE TRUSTED PEDIATRICIAN

"Since PANDAS is associated with strep throat, you can bring Cody in without an appointment for a rapid strep test if you feel he needs it," Dr. Meneely said during the follow-up appointment. "And I recommend you see the child psychiatrist at Vanderbilt Children's Psychiatric Hospital next. He'll be able to help you with CBT—that's cognitive behavioral therapy—and with Zoloft."

With that, Liz and Cody left their pediatrician's office. She still did not understand why Cody would have to take antidepressants for strep, but Liz trusted Dr. Meneely. A seasoned doctor who had been in practice for over thirty years—at least ten of which Liz had been bringing Kelsey and Cody to him—the man never seemed to be in a hurry, and he was always smiling.

Liz was confident he would be able to help her put together this PANDAS puzzle.

BUT FIRST, OFF TO LIZ'S PSYCHIATRIST

Cody had not left his mother's side since he had been released from the hospital.

A few days later, Liz needed to go to an appointment with Dr. Asher, the psychiatrist she had been seeing since the divorce. Cody insisted on going with her.

"See? I'm ready!" Cody crammed his feet into his tennis shoes keeping his eyes on her as if she were going to try to escape without him. His panic-stricken face convinced her to bring him along.

Once they were settled in Dr. Asher's office, Liz handed Cody a Rubik's Cube to try and keep him occupied while she and her doctor discussed the various symptoms she was being treated for, each of which had a different prescription medication—Klonopin for when she felt anxious, Vyvanse for focus, Flexeril to help lessen her nighttime teeth grinding.

Dr. Asher picked up, though, that there was more going on than just the stress related to a divorce. "Is there something else you're not telling me?" she asked. "You seem anxious."

"Well, yes," Liz admitted. "It seems like Cody has PANDAS, and I'm supposed to get Zoloft from a doctor who can't see him for six months, and he's supposed to be getting CBT, and I don't even really know what CBT is!"

Even just saying it all felt exhausting.

"That would be overwhelming even without everything else you've been dealing with the past couple of years! We can talk through how this is affecting you," Dr. Asher assured Liz. "We also have a child psychiatrist who may be able to help. You can ask her all the questions you want."

Liz smiled. "*That* is the best medication you could have given me!" She felt relieved to leave the office with an appointment on the books for Cody.

NOTHING MAKES HIM COMFORTABLE

Liz was doing everything the doctors said, but something was still wrong with Cody. Nothing seemed to make her son feel comfortable—not the thickest socks, softest pillow, or the warmest soup. He was anxious and had trouble sleeping. The dilated pupils, paranoia, and crawling spiders were gone, but his OCD had not gone anywhere.

Liz took Cody back to Dr. Meneely's office for a rapid strep test to see if that was the problem, but the test came back negative. Dr. Meneely had not drawn any blood, which confused Liz. Still, she trusted their long-term pediatrician's medical judgment and deferred. She was hopeful that the appointment with a child psychiatrist would bring answers as to why Cody was not one hundred percent yet.

CHILD PSYCHIATRY AND COGNITIVE BEHAVIORAL THERAPY

After listening to the child psychiatrist trying to explain PANDAS, Liz asked, "So, whatever the anti-DNase B messed up, the CBT will fix?"

"That is the theory," she answered confidently. "Let's go ahead and have you guys meet the therapist. She specializes in children with autism and is excellent."

Horrified, Liz asked, "Is PANDAS autism?"

"It's a form of autism, yes. It's on the extreme end of the scale."

Extreme end of the autism scale? What?

The words felt like a blow to her gut. In a daze, she followed the psychiatrist across the hallway. Before she even caught her breath, let alone process this new label, Cody's CBT session had been scheduled for the following week.

Liz pushed autism out of her mind and focused on the CBT, which was going well. The whole family, including John, took turns attending sessions with Cody. The therapist guided each one of them on ways to help tame what she referred to as "the OCD monster."

NO MORE ZOLOFT

Meanwhile, Cody did not like the side effects of Zoloft, saying that it made him feel weird. The child psychiatrist had mentioned that if it did not make that much of a difference, he could stop taking it.

Cody seems hollow, a shell of my former son.

With the doctor's permission, she took him off Zoloft.

COMPLEX REGIONAL PAIN SYNDROME

For nearly ten years, Liz had been bothered by the reminder of those awful boils on her eyelid. As her birthday gift to herself, she went to see Dr. Charles—a plastic surgeon who had formerly served as medical director at the spa—about an eyelift.

"We have been through a lot, and I really need to do something for myself," Liz explained.

Over the years, Dr. Charles had been both a mentor and a friend. They shared many mutual clients, so he was aware of what was transpiring in Liz's world.

"Yes, you do," he affirmed. "I'm so sorry for everything you have been going through with John and now Cody. The eyelift will help, but what else is going on with you?"

"What do you mean?"

"Your fingers," he answered. "They're clubbing."

Liz looked at her hands. Dr. Charles was right. Her knuckles looked different than before, as did her fingernails. She had noticed that the veins in her right hand looked larger lately, but that was hardly anything to see a doctor about.

Since Liz was comfortable talking with Dr. Charles, she went on to explain all the weird things that she had recently experienced, including the wrist pain and numbness that she had been trying to ignore for months.

"Just last week," she added, "my wrist completely locked up."

Dr. Charles scribbled down something on a piece of paper and handed it to her. "Look into this," he prompted her.

Complex regional pain syndrome/CRPS, the note read.

"You should probably see a neurologist—perhaps a rheumatologist also."

Her mind began to race.

My focus has always been on Cody. I don't have time for there to be something wrong with me!

She wanted to get to the bottom of it so she could get on with her life.

It only took a few hours of looking into CRPS before she recognized all the symptoms as her own. After learning that this syndrome was associated with an injury or surgery it all fit. Three years earlier, Liz had broken a small bone in her right pinky finger which had refused to heal even after surgery.

According to the doctor, the pain Liz described had been much worse than it should have been and, ultimately, the solution had been to fuse the bone. Liz had just blindly agreed with what the doctors recommended.

In hindsight, it seemed like that was when the CRPS started.

If she indeed had CRPS, and if it had been spreading, then Dr. Charles was right—she needed to get to these other doctors.

How could her orthopedic doctors and surgeons have missed that?

The literature described it as one of the most painful syndromes known to humankind, and although she read that there was no cure for it, she simply would not believe that ending up disabled or committing suicide because of the physical pain—nine hundred times more common among CRPS sufferers—could be her fate.

Liz stared at her once-beautiful, agile hands. She thought of the times they spent in the catcher's mitt fielding softballs for Kelsey, the days at the piano practicing Bach's *Solfeggietto* to perfection, and the hours carefully tying the sweetest, tiniest bow onto each of the Christmas cards she had sent out just the year before...

And now her hands were—as Dr. Charles pointed out—clubbing?

Would I get to experience such treasured moments again? Worse yet, this could end my career.

Liz was not prepared to accept some debilitating, horrifically painful disease that resulted in mangled hands. She went to see a neurologist who said she did not have carpal tunnel issues, but he prescribed Lyrica for the nerve pain. She also went to see a rheumatologist who could find no explanation for her symptoms. Next, Liz consulted her orthopedist to see if he had any ideas.

If only he had caught this, it could have been treated.

He felt terrible, but all he could do was to recommend she went to a physical therapist and a chiropractor.

After several weeks of various treatments, Liz still awoke in the same state of pain and numbness each morning as she had been in before. Meanwhile, her jaw was getting tighter, and the burning pain in her neck was relentless.

When she went to see Dr. Charles for her eye procedure, he suggested that she see a pain specialist, which she did.

"Really? I don't want to be on pain meds forever," she told the pain specialist. "Is there anything else we could try?"

"Well," he said, "we could try nerve blocks."

If the procedure worked, it would block the nerves from conducting pain, and Liz indeed might not have to take pain medication.

NOT MY HAIR!

Maybe Liz was moving to stage two of CRPS. She began losing her hair to an extraordinary degree. Her research pointed her to a product called Nioxin. She immediately purchased the entire system.

I will not *lose my hair! I can't be a bald spa owner with clubbed hands.*

After just a few weeks of using the system, Liz's hair started looking thicker. This made her feel better. It was also oddly comforting to know that at stage three of CRPS, the hair loss would stop.

Another symptom was muscle shrinkage. To combat that, Liz increased her workouts to seven days a week.

THE OCD MONSTER

After the completion of a nerve block procedure, Liz was able to bend her wrist again. She was delighted. Between this procedure, some nonsteroidal anti-inflammatory treatments, Nioxin, and her workouts, Liz felt more confident that she could go on with her life as planned.

She couldn't wait to show her children the results when they walked in the door.

When Michelle asked about her hand, Liz joyfully wriggled it in the air. "Awesome, Mom!" Michelle smiled.

Cody followed, giving her an approving nod. As he headed toward his room, Adam trudged in through the front door. Something seemed to be bothering him. Liz asked what was wrong.

"Cody made fun of me on the bus."

"Cody," Liz called. "Come back here. We need to talk."

"Mom, it's just that Adam wears that same jacket every day even though I've told him over and over that it's tacky." He was exasperated. "He needs to wear that new jacket Dad bought him."

In almost nine months of CBT, Cody had acquired various "tools" to help him deal with issues that arose, one of which was to talk about the "OCD monster."

"Cody, is this about Adam's jacket," she asked, "or is this more of the OCD monster trying to take control?"

The approach did not help one bit. Cody simply shrugged.

STRESS AMONG THE SIBLINGS

Cody relentlessly followed Adam around the house, offering a constant stream of unsolicited advice. Michelle had no tolerance for Cody and avoided him at all costs.

It hurt Liz deeply to watch her children so divided.

This wasn't the way things were supposed to be. It's not the way things were.

Adam became more withdrawn, so Liz encouraged the boys to do activities together. She ventured upstairs to see if she could lure Adam out of his room. Cracking open the door to his bedroom, she found him playing a video game again.

Liz had taken his computer away for weeks at a time, lectured, grounded him, and yelled, but nothing shook him from his wild idea that he could earn a million dollars from other people paying to watch him play video games on YouTube.

"Did you turn in those assignments that we did last night?" she wanted to know.

Despite her having reminded him right before school, Adam still forgot.

"How come?"

He shrugged his shoulders.

She raised her voice. "I just can't understand!"

"I forgot."

This back and forth would continue until it became so frustrating that it simply was not worth the effort to try to talk with him. Liz decided that it was time for her and Adam to meet with the CBT therapist.

COGNITIVE BEHAVIORAL THERAPY: FAIL

The therapist concluded that Adam was falling into the victim role with Cody as the aggressor and that a pattern of codependency was developing.

Codependent? Adam tries as hard as he can to get away from Cody!

It was easy for the therapist to give it a name but teaching Adam what this meant and how to deal with it was another matter that Liz was not prepared or equipped to tackle.

After reading up on codependency, Liz summed it up for Adam: "When it comes to Cody, you have to draw firm boundaries."

Not agreeing with much of the therapist's approach, Liz felt like a boundary was imminent on that front. She maintained her civility with the therapist, but on the inside, Liz was slowly coming undone.

The CBT worked occasionally. But most of the time, it was a miserable failure.

CHAPTER 3

Trying to Get Help

FALL 2011

That summer, Liz had planned as many outings for the family as she could. But Cody's newly acquired OCD caused the children to constantly argue in public.

Once school was back in full swing, Cody developed an annoyance with crowds. He was constantly fidgeting and could not sit still for but a few minutes.

He had also been feeling a little sick to his stomach, but the CBT therapist said it was probably nerves.

Getting Cody to go to church became a stressful event and trying to force him only made things worse. To simplify things, the Harris family started having church at home on Sunday mornings. This worked well, especially since it allowed Cody to play his guitar while they all sang along.

A few weeks into this new arrangement, while they were singing, Cody stopped playing in the middle of the song.

"Mom, my stomach hurts again," he said.

This is not nerves. Cody is completely relaxed, doing what he loves.

Liz knew she had to do something. He was getting worse, so she thought it would be a good idea to get another anti-DNase B test to see what his number was.

Liz did not trust the rapid strep test; she was adamant to get his blood drawn.

If Cody could have another anti-DNase B test, they will know if the number of strep antibodies had changed.

She scheduled an appointment with Dr. Meneely. Their pediatrician would not administer the test despite Liz offering to pay out of pocket.

All he has to do is order it!

She tried harder. "If you could test him now and then again in a few weeks, we will know if his titers are rising," she insisted. "If they are, it means he has an active strep infection—like the last time his stomach hurt this badly—and he can get antibiotics because, as you know, strep doesn't just go away on its own."

"Vanderbilt Hospital will have to order that test," Dr. Meneely smiled.

Why won't he order this test? The last bill from the hospital visit was $27,000! Does he want me to drive to the hospital and pay thousands of dollars for a proper strep test?

She tried to remain calm and salvage the appointment. "Well, I saw on the PANDAS website that they recommended putting children on a low dose of penicillin for the long term to prevent future strep infections."

Dr. Meneely simply shook his head and kept smiling. "No," he insisted. "Antibiotics are *not* a good idea."

What could be better than protecting Cody's brain from strep exposure?

Cody explained to his doctor that he could not eat. Dr. Meneely explained that ADHD medications could sometimes cause a decreased appetite. The pediatrician turned his gaze back to Liz, "Let's change the Concerta to Adderall."

Changing Cody's meds hasn't fixed anything. Could we just entertain the idea for one second that Cody may be ill? If these medications can lead to decreased appetite, we would have seen a consistent pattern not months of normal appetite then two weeks of no appetite. Simply changing his meds does not make sense.

Against her better judgment, Liz kept quiet and took the useless prescription he handed her.

DILATED PUPILS

It had been nearly two years since John had moved out and moved on. John picked the kids up for a Friday night visit. When he brought them home, he was beaming.

"Cody was amazing," John told Liz. "He jammed on the guitar with one of my friends for three hours tonight." John stood in the doorway while the children filed into the house. "He was *so* intense. I've never seen him like that."

But after John left, Liz noticed that Cody did not seem well. His pupils were dilated, he had dark circles under his eyes, and he was agitated. At the same time, he was nauseated, lethargic, and looked like he might pass out.

Cody slumped down against the wall in the bathroom with Rusty at his side.

"Mom, the songs keep playing in my head over and over! I can't shut them out."

Were the auditory hallucinations starting again?

A few hours later, Cody finally felt calm enough to sleep.

CLENCHED FISTS, STIFF BODY, LOTS OF PAIN

The next morning, John picked them up for breakfast and a playdate with Susie's kids. John and Susie had been dating for over a year, and Liz was thankful that the kids all got along well.

Within a few hours, John called explaining that Cody was not feeling well at all. He brought the kids back to Liz's home.

Liz got Cody settled into bed, but he could not relax. "Whenever I move my head hurts," he moaned.

She put a cool towel across Cody's forehead, but he did not want anyone touching him nor could he stand any light. His fists were clenched, every muscle in his body was stiff and he was in a tremendous amount of pain.

This time, Liz recorded a video on her phone so she could show Dr. Meneely. Then she called John to hear what could have led to Cody's current state.

"I think he just ate too much for breakfast," John suggested.

"Dammit, John! This isn't from overeating. I am taking Cody to the hospital!"

John reminded Liz that they were still paying the bill from when Cody had been admitted and asked her to reconsider a trip to the emergency room. She reluctantly conceded.

Liz had barely wrapped up the conversation with John when Cody projectile-vomited several times.

Since taking Cody to the hospital had been vetoed, she was more determined than ever to get Dr. Meneely's help. That weekend, she sent him an email with the video clips of Cody and included an excerpt from a book by Kenneth Bock, MD, a functional medicine doctor who suggests that childhood pneumonia—as Cody often had since he was a baby—was tied to PANDAS.

Liz had a hunch that these were important pieces of the puzzle.

GETTING FED-UP FIGHTING THE SYSTEM

By the end of that week, Liz had not yet heard from Dr. Meneely, and Cody still was not feeling well. She called his office to follow up, wanting to know if Dr. Meneely had watched the videos she had sent.

The nurse dodged the question, suggesting instead that if Cody exhibited the kind of behavior portrayed in the videos again, Liz should take him to the emergency room.

"So that they can change his ADHD medication, add Zoloft again, and charge us another $27,000?!" Liz was fed-up with having to fight the system, but she was not about to give up.

The nurse referred her to a child neurologist, admitting that the waiting list was six months long.

"Cody doesn't have six months to wait! Plus, the primary care physician is the one who's supposed to test for strep and prescribe antibiotics for kids with PANDAS!" Liz objected.

The nurse gave Liz three more physicians' names. One was no longer in practice, the second was not taking new patients, and the third had never heard of PANDAS.

According to stories shared by other moms on a Facebook page for parents of children with PANDAS, they were not having any more success getting answers than she was.

Liz was tempted to find Cody another doctor, but it had been a doctor at *that* practice who had recognized the symptoms of PANDAS from a three-minute description over the phone a year ago.

Liz decided to stay put. Maybe Dr. Meneely knew what he was doing.

PRESSING PAUSE ON COGNITIVE BEHAVIORAL THERAPY

It was time for Cody's weekly CBT appointment, but because he was so sick, Liz convinced the therapist to drive to their house to see for herself.

At this point, Cody had attended almost thirty therapy sessions, and even though Liz had done everything the therapist suggested—including taking guitar lessons to inspire creativity, encouraging his physical fitness with jujitsu classes, and supporting him on the wrestling team—Cody's erratic behaviors continued.

After seeing how physically sick the twelve-year-old was, the therapist insisted that medical rule-outs were needed before Cody continued with talk therapy.

I wish she *could call Dr. Meneely and explain that!*

HELD HOSTAGE BY A SYSTEM

Cody's symptoms improved with no rhyme or reason. But just as he mysteriously improved, Cody would start having strange symptoms again out of the blue.

About six weeks later, Cody started rearranging pillows again, but Dr. Meneely did not feel he needed to be seen. But when Cody started waking up at four in the morning, struggling to catch his breath, Liz insisted, and Dr. Meneely agreed.

He read over the notes from the intake nurse. "Hmm... could be anxiety disorder... or it may be asthma," he mused.

Maybe he doesn't know what he is doing.

"We can send him to a psychologist if this persists," the doctor concluded.

He already goes to one! She won't even see him again until a medical doctor figures out what is wrong with my child. This is a lung problem. Why would you even consider sending him to a psychologist *when he cannot breathe?*

Her son needed help, but Liz's hands were tied. She felt like she was being held hostage by Dr. Meneely. She had made a few phone calls to other pediatricians only to learn they did not know how to treat PANDAS either. She was fighting the system and did not stand a chance.

She could not order the labs Cody needed herself nor could she write the prescriptions for antibiotics even if she had the lab results.

I'm helpless.

TWO STEPS FORWARD, ONE STEP BACK

Unexpectedly, Cody's physical condition seemed to improve again and by Christmas, the Harris family had an enjoyable holiday. The kids went back to school in January.

But it did not take long for Liz to receive an email from one of his teachers explaining that Cody exhibited some behavioral challenges. For no apparent reason, he ran down the hall flailing his arms wildly.

Cody's not in kindergarten, he's in the seventh grade! What is going on?

Within the month, Cody's unusual behaviors escalated rapidly. After he received four bus referrals in a single week, all for things that made absolutely no sense, she decided that it was in everyone's best interest for her to keep him home.

CHAPTER 4

Flares

NOTHING WORKS

It had been thirteen months since the first hospital visit that started the PANDAS nightmare, and with their pediatrician not willing to order the test, Liz continued with her own research. She learned that what Cody was experiencing were referred to as *flares*.

Flares occurred when Cody's OCD and related behaviors were activated during a strep infection.

Once she had a name for it, she started paying closer attention to the cycles. There seemed to be no rhyme or reason for when the flares came and went nor for how long they lasted. What was clear, though, is that there were a lot of ups and downs.

Cody's flares gave off the same kind of energy as a Metallica concert about to take place.

The first several days or weeks of a flare was like the five o'clock crowd shuffling in for the seven o'clock concert—low-level activity and a bit of anticipation but no feeling of urgency. The spectators

33

can sense something big is about to take place but are not sure exactly what.

During the next phase of his flare, the anxiety and excitement heighten. It is as if more fans arrive and start pushing and shoving to vie for the perfect seat.

In the final scene, the band explodes on stage with music blaring and strobe lights flashing. Lit joints, fizzy beers, and screaming fans overtake the scene. No security firm can control the crowd. Those who try risk the outburst of an enraged mob.

The aftermath looked different for a flare than for a heavy metal concert. A show winds down rather abruptly, leaving the band and the fans stoked yet exhausted. But a flare takes between a week or two to fizzle out and leaves all parties bone-weary.

Even when Cody was not flaring, there was still some degree of clean up from the last "concert."

And during the flares, any tools she used to manage the erratic behaviors were a waste of time. Keeping him at home seemed to be her only option.

Liz contacted his teachers and arranged to get Cody's work by email. All assignments were completed and turned in on time, so it was hard to understand when she received a phone call from the principal. "We need to have a meeting to discuss Cody's absences."

A DOCTOR'S NOTE, PLEASE

Liz and John were told that they needed a doctor's note to excuse Cody for his excessive school absenteeism. Without a note, they had to send Cody back to school or Liz would be charged with truancy.

She reached out to Dr. Meneely's office but never heard back. She had no choice but to send Cody to school—her being jailed for truancy would not help any of her children. Incensed, she made it clear to the principal that sending Cody back to school was not a good idea on any level.

A MEETING AT THE PRINCIPAL'S OFFICE

Merely three days later, the principal called and insisted Liz come to the school right away. She knew that Cody had no "stop switch" at this point and dreaded finding out what had happened.

"Ms. Harris, it seems that Cody has put a laxative in another child's drink at lunch." The principal crossed his arms, but relief washed over Liz.

It could have been worse.

"We aren't going to charge him with a class B felony," the principal continued as if he were doing her a big favor. "But we are suspending him for ten days."

A felony?! He's only twelve years old!

She had repeatedly told the school officials that Cody should not be at school in his condition. She felt that the school had gotten off easy, that things could have been worse. Determined not to come unglued in front of her son, Liz stood up. "We need to leave before I say something I may regret."

On the way home, she grilled Cody for what he had done. "Those were Rusty's prescription laxatives, and there was only one left!"

She was exasperated, yet relieved that Cody would have the ten days at home he needed for the flare to calm down.

GETTING A DOCTOR'S NOTE

Liz did not want to be threatened with jail for truancy, should this happen again.

During the suspension, Liz reached out to Dr. Meneely's office multiple times. Finally, she received a phone call from the receptionist advising her that the note was ready. It simply read: "Cody Harris is currently under my care for a disease resulting from streptococcal illness."

Liz's trust in their doctor was slightly restored.

She had resolved to fire Dr. Meneely, but she did not know where else to take Cody. Besides, if he believed that Cody had an illness resulting from a streptococcal infection, then surely, he understood the nature of the illness he was treating.

Maybe I need to trust him to do his job while I focus even harder on mine: being a good parent.

ANOTHER DIAGNOSIS

Liz was committed to making sure the other kids were doing well. She took Michelle and Adam to Mission Clinic for their wellness checks.

Mission is a Christian clinic where the kids had been going for years. Having had plenty of stress in their lives, Liz chose to keep them with Dr. Brunner, their childhood pediatrician, rather than moving their care to someone closer to home.

Dr. Brunner was kind and seemed to genuinely care about the kids. Both Michelle and Adam were struggling to focus at school, so their pediatrician suggested starting them on Adderall for attention deficit disorder (ADD).

Liz was perplexed by this new diagnosis.

How is it that all my kids have either ADD or ADHD? I have ADHD, so I can understand that Cody and Kelsey could take after me. But now my adopted kids have ADD? That seems strange!

Each new issue that arose was far from being a mystery of its own. It was all part of one big puzzle.

But Liz had no way of knowing that at the time.

OFF TO A WRESTLING MEET

With Adderall, hard work, and support, Michelle brought her grades up quickly, but Adam still lagged in his schoolwork.

One Saturday morning after breakfast, the rest of the family headed to a wrestling meet to watch Cody compete. Liz insisted that Adam stay home to work on completing several outstanding assignments. Adam seemed relieved.

Sitting at those meets for eight hours on a Saturday was not something Liz looked forward to, either, but Cody had made it to the finals, and she was happy to support his efforts.

Cody had no prior wrestling experience, yet he won all his matches that day, leading to a match against the state champion. Cody was winning before being penalized for an illegal move. The referee had him start on his back, and as he was resisting his opponent, something went wrong.

Liz could see her son's face turn gray. The referee immediately stopped the match. It looked like Cody's left collarbone was broken.

Within thirty minutes, the Harrises were in the emergency room at Vanderbilt Hospital.

There, Liz learned how unusual it is for a collarbone to splinter from resistance. "This type of injury usually results from something like a high-speed car wreck," a doctor explained.

Cody's trophy for his wrestling match? A metal plate supporting his shattered bone.

CHAPTER 5

Imperfect Parenting

DETERMINED TO GET HELP

Liz was up late one night reviewing the products to be used in a new facial at the spa. The television was on, and an infomercial caught her attention. It offered concrete tools to change a child's behavior and restore peace to the family. The program was called the Total Transformation.

Liz placed an order and signed up for online support.

Nobody had ever told Liz she wasn't being a good mother, but the looks she was given had said it all.

Once the materials arrived, she dove in headfirst. She was able to put a name to several behaviors she had seen in Cody, and there were also some she hadn't seen.

She was desperate for answers and although this program was a lot to implement, she was determined to give it everything she had.

IMPLEMENTING TOTAL TRANSFORMATION

Liz appreciated that this program seemed to remove the emotional piece from disciplining the children. As suggested, the Harris family started having regular family meetings.

At one such meeting, Liz launched her plan for what the program called "empowered parenting." She explained the official new house rules and posted them on the refrigerator.

Since the spa vied for her attention, Liz hired a general manager so she could focus on being a full-time mother for a while. After all, her children were more important than the business.

It felt good to have a plan, a system, and a helpline that supported her in her parenting. In fact, Liz called the support line so much that she was on a first-name basis with several of the operators.

REWARDS AND CONSEQUENCES

"Remember, we all agreed that it was fair to clean up after ourselves," Liz explained as she filled out a ticket for a demerit. "We're all part of this family, and each member has to contribute."

Liz was even more zealous in acknowledging good behavior. "Adam, you were kind to Cody," she said as she proudly presented him with a point card as a reward.

On Fridays, she met with each child to tally their weekly points and demerits and to hand out weekend rewards or consequences.

Liz enjoyed parenting this way. She felt more confident when she had rules covering every possibility and a proven, no-nonsense protocol to follow. It gave her a newfound hope and a sense of security in dealing with her children.

She could feel confident that Cody's misbehaviors were not from any lack of parenting skills on her part.

Although Cody was trying as hard as Michelle and Adam—if not harder—he could only make it for a few hours at a time without a demerit. He just could not hold it together long enough to earn a reward.

It did not feel right for Cody to never earn enough points, so Liz rewarded him for trying. She knew his heart; he simply could not seem to control his behavior. She decided to trust the process and press forward with the program.

Part of being a good parent is spending quality time with your children, so Liz set aside Sunday evenings to read to them, Wednesday nights for family meetings, and one night on the weekend for games.

NATURAL CONSEQUENCES

Another aspect of the perfect parenting program was to provide support to the administrators of the school. Liz scheduled a meeting with the assistant principal and requested to be notified anytime there was an issue with Cody.

During Cody's eighth-grade school year, Liz visited the school twenty-seven times.

Cody needed to understand the consequences of his actions, so Liz vowed to fully support the administration in their efforts to discipline her son according to school policy. Natural consequences, after all, was something that the Total Transformation system encouraged, and Liz was committed to perfect adherence.

However, during a meeting near the end of the school year, the assistant principal took it to the next level. "Cody, if you refuse to follow the rules, the school will have to file unruly charges and you will have to appear in front of a judge."

Liz's eyes got big.

Was being taken to appear before a judge the next "natural consequence"? What else can I do to stop things from getting worse?!

She had already exhausted all the in-home discipline options she could think of in addition to the ones recommended by Total Transformation. These behaviors had no logic, and logical discipline was not working.

MORE HANDS ON DECK

Despite having a general manager at the spa, Liz's business demanded her attention. And as the kids got older, they also seemed to need more of Liz's time, especially to take them everywhere they needed to go.

Liz hired Miss Maria to help with the cleaning once a week and asked Mark—a handyman, who had been helping her as needed around the house for years—to work full time.

Mark was an unassuming guy who rarely got rattled and had gotten to know the children fairly well. Liz appreciated his calm demeanor, especially when life got crazy. Mark agreed to help Liz run the kids here and there—like a nanny would—as well as take care of general maintenance. Liz called him their "maintenance manny."

Having Mark on staff was a saving grace as Cody's behavior was becoming more bizarre by the moment. Liz urgently needed backup. And with Cody officially being a teenager, learning from Mark how to fix things could be good for him.

CREATING SAFE SPACES

Liz could not seem to find things around the house lately. She opened the cabinet to an empty space where the canned goods used to be.

Has Miss Maria been working on overdrive?

"Where are all the green beans?" she called out.

"I saw Cody taking them up to the attic," Michelle offered.

"The *attic?*" Liz went to see for herself.

Sure enough, a collection of supplies sat near the attic window. She checked other out-of-the-way areas and discovered that Cody had created small stashes in the attic, crawl space, and basement. He had also installed deadbolts on the inside of the closet.

She rescued her green beans, cases of water, brooms, and a host of other items and asked Cody why he was doing that.

"In case we get attacked," he explained. "We have to be prepared." The fact that Cody felt the need to create safe spaces concerned her deeply, but when she noticed that he had also added toy guns that he had spray-painted black, she called John for help.

"Oh, that's completely normal," he dismissed her concern. "All boys play with guns."

"But John, aren't you the one who just sent me an article about Grant Acord, that boy in Oregon who got sentenced to ten years in juvenile detention for planning an attack on his school? Remember, he had PANDAS too."

"Grant's mother said that she wasn't able to get the right medical treatment for her son and the OCD had turned into something far worse."

Liz desperately wanted to avoid something worse.

There were too many similarities between Cody and Grant to be ignored. Grant was seventeen when the incident took place, so she figured she had about four years to make sure Cody was well and did not follow the same path.

Liz was determined to get medical treatment much sooner than that, though. She decided to continue her pursuit of antibiotics to treat the strep, prevent future infections, and in doing so, put a stop to these bizarre behaviors.

THE NATURAL CONSEQUENCES OF BEING EXPOSED TO STREP

Miss Maria was waiting for her when she got off a call with her mother. "Ms. Liz," she said, "I am sorry, but my throat hurts so badly that I cannot finish cleaning your house today. I have to go home."

"That's fine, Maria. I hope you feel better soon." Liz held her breath, hoping it was just a sore throat, but when Maria let her know that she had a strep test done and it was positive, Liz braced herself.

Nonononono!

Cody was especially close to Maria, and she occasionally helped him with his Spanish homework.

I hope Cody hasn't caught it!

A few days later, the school nurse called. "Ms. Harris, Cody just threw up. You should come and pick him up."

Terror gripped Liz.

By the time Liz got to the school, she noticed changes not only in his behavior but also in his appearance. He looked kind of scary, almost savage—tougher, his face was tense—not like a thirteen-year-old child.

"Mom, what time are we leaving for the surgeon?" he demanded.

Liz had scheduled an appointment to have a cyst removed that had appeared above Cody's left knee a few months earlier. "We aren't going—you are sick."

"What?" Cody's eyes locked onto her face. "I'm not sick."

Cody walked toward her with a look of defiance that she had never seen before. This did not seem like Cody at all.

Liz recognized what the Total Transformation materials described as oppositional defiant disorder (ODD).

I've been implementing this program for almost a year. How can things be getting worse?!

This had come on overnight. Cody had never talked to his mom like this before.

Turn over another piece of the puzzle.

"Cody, you're scaring me," she exclaimed. "I need to tell you something. Miss Maria just told me that she had strep."

Shaken by this news, Cody came out of whatever seemed to have overtaken him and apologized.

THE LAST STRAW

Cody's remorse did not last, though. Liz was at her wit's end. She watched as he slipped further away from his mom and deeper into his own world. To try and connect, she called the kids down to work on homework.

Michelle and Adam came right away. Cody strolled downstairs about ten minutes later in his bathrobe. Within minutes, Cody started slithering around like a snake, first on the couch, then on the floor.

Liz had had it. "Cody, that's so disrespectful! If you can't sit up and act right, we are all going to get dressed and go to the library." She knew that was the last thing Cody wanted to do, but he kept rolling around on the floor until she had no other choice but to make good on her threat.

"Everyone get dressed; we are going to the library."

Cody gave his mother a defiant no.

"No? Did you just tell me no, young man?" She had thoroughly discussed scenarios like this with the professionals at the Total Transformation support hotline. They had told her several times that involving law enforcement was the next step. Liz had heard this same message from the assistant principal and now from experts in transforming children's behavior.

She desperately did not want to take this step, but Cody's future was in her hands. She would follow the advice of people with much more training and experience than she had.

"Cody, either you get dressed to go to the library, or you get dressed to go to juvenile hall."

Cody turned and went upstairs.

Thank goodness!

CALLING THE POLICE

"Are you ready, guys?" Liz called, ready to head out.

"I'm not going to the library," Cody declared.

"Then why are you dressed?"

"I'm going to juvenile hall."

"What?!" Liz could not believe it. "No, Cody. You do *not* want to do that," she pleaded.

"Yes, I do," he answered, staring her down. "Call them."

If I don't call the police now, Cody will never take me seriously.

So, Liz called the police.

When the officer arrived, Liz told her son he still had a choice—either go with his family or go with the police. Cody was determined to go with the police.

The officer told Liz she had to sign a petition for unruly behavior. She was also told that once Cody went to court, the petition would likely be dropped.

After some discussion, the officer agreed it was for the best that they took Cody. "That usually gives them enough of a scare," he told Liz, assuring her that juvenile detention was for children and was nothing like adult jail.

Liz signed the papers. Tears streamed down her face when the car pulled away.

This could end up being a good thing for Cody. If this is a behavioral issue, maybe this could fix it. But if they also think it's is a medical issue, maybe this will help us get a court order from the judge that would force Dr. Meneely to order Cody the anti-DNase B titer test so we can prove he has PANDAS.

YOU CALLED THE POLICE? A NOTE FROM THE AUTHOR

I am taking the liberty to interrupt the story and add an editorial comment. I have been asked countless times why I called the police on my son. I have cut so much of the story so far to make it more palpable to you, the reader. Hence, you may also be wondering why I would call the cops.

I had pressure from every angle daily to do something about Cody's behavior. I was out of ideas. The mere thought of my child doing something that would cost him or others their lives kept me on this relentless quest to find out what was really going on.

It was my understanding that the juvenile detention center was a place that helped children when all else had failed. I erroneously believed that there were therapists, medical professionals, educators, and the like who would all be available in these types of places.

During flares, I witnessed Cody do things that he would never do otherwise. During those times, he seemed to have absolutely no ability to stop himself. They were compulsions.

The kid in Oregon who had PANDAS and who also had no doctor willing to treat him ended up with a ten-year sentence! I was not going just sit idly and watch this same thing happen to Cody.

Okay. Back to the story...

SOMETHING IS VERY WRONG

Liz soon got a message from John. "I understand that you called the cops on Cody. I wish that you would've called me instead."

There was no mincing words when Liz responded. "Something is *very* wrong with our son, and I'm afraid of what he might end up doing. I don't want to have to live with the guilt of not having done more to stop whatever this is."

"Either Cody needs consistent boundaries, or there's something far more to this PANDAS than either of us understand," she continued. "Besides, both Total Transformation *and* the officer confirmed that the goal of the juvenile detention system is to help children who go there! Plus, it could help us get a court order, and then Dr. Meneely will have no choice but to order Cody the anti-DNase B test.

IN-HOME DETENTION

The next morning, John and Liz attended the detention hearing. It had only been one night, but Liz felt like it had been ten years since she had seen her son. Cody stood beside them in his blue prison attire as John tried to explain PANDAS and ask for a test to be ordered to confirm, but the judge looked at him and Liz like they had three heads.

Liz did not get the chance to say a single word before being handed a list of rules for what they called in-home detention. She had to make sure Cody followed these, or *she* would be held in contempt of court and be sent to jail for ten days.

As Liz reviewed the paper, her heart sank. She had implemented most of these things as consequences for years, and more recently she had taken them to a whole other level with Total Transformation.

There was not anything on that list she had not already tried multiple times. If it had worked, why were they in court that day? Liz was heartbroken.

I don't need more rules. I need a medical test. Nobody even asked what we've tried!

FILING A PETITION

Later that day, Liz contacted the assistant principal due to Cody's absence related to their court appearance, and they discussed the situation.

Since Cody's behaviors were as unpredictable at school as Liz described them to be at home, they both agreed that providing documentation of Cody's illogical behaviors at school may help the judge make a better decision.

So, the assistant principal submitted the documentation.

If the judge could see that these behaviors were consistent both at home and school, he could understand that this is a medical issue, not a parental one. Surely, if the judge had all the information, he could make a more informed decision at the next hearing and help Cody get the test to prove that he is sick—not simply unruly.

BACK TO THE DETENTION CENTER AND COURT

It was Liz's forty-first birthday, but the last thing she felt like doing was to celebrate. She sat at her computer reviewing spa-related emails when Adam rushed over.

"Mom, Cody just held me down," he explained. Adam was crying and beet red. "He did a jujitsu move on me."

Cody was quick to justify. "Adam wouldn't stop playing my keyboard even though I asked him over and over again not to."

Regardless of the reason, Cody knew better than to use jujitsu moves on his brother. This was just another in a series of aggressive behaviors.

The last thing Cody needed to see was his mother breaking the law. He was standing right there when the judge threatened John and Liz within an inch of their lives. Hence, per the court's order, Liz drove her son to the detention center and explained that he had broken the rules. She was also hoping that her son's growing aggression would cool a little if he spent a night at the center.

The court system was backed up, though, so Cody had to spend three nights away before his court appearance. But for the assistant principal to get the documentation in front of the judge, she had to file a petition. This was the third petition within two weeks. Hence, the judge appointed Melinda Ledford, guardian *ad litem*,[4] to investigate the situation.

It worked! We have been assigned our very own guardian to help us with Cody!

DETENTION = A JAIL FOR CHILDREN

Relieved to have a child specialist involved in their case, Liz tried to get to know Ms. Ledford a little while waiting for Cody to be released.

Ms. Ledford had another appointment and had to leave, so Liz wandered over and looked through the door and down the hallway that led to the detention center. Something did not seem right.

---

4   Not her real name. A guardian *ad litem* is an attorney appointed by the court on behalf of a minor. They are tasked with making sure the best interest of the child is protected.

She asked one of the guards if she could have a tour of the detention center. When the officer acted a little concerned, Liz became suspicious and insisted.

At the end of the long hallway, there were cells with metal bunk beds and guards. This horrified Liz. Learning that there were *no* professionals available to provide therapy for the youth and that Cody had been incarcerated like he was a criminal? It mortified her.

Once Liz had Cody safely in the car, she called her psychiatrist, Dr. Asher. "I know you don't treat children, but you know more about Cody's case than anyone else! Please help us. There's no way I can let Cody go back to that awful place ever again. Can you help us, please?!"

Dr. Asher agreed to take him on as a patient. After assessing him, she prescribed an atypical antipsychotic drug, an anti-anxiety medication, and a mood stabilizer in addition to his Adderall.

Although Liz did not like the idea of so many medications, she would do anything to keep him from having to go back to detention. If it meant he had to take all these meds, so be it.

CALLING 911

But the early warning signs of a flare had already occurred, and that Friday night, when the children arrived home from John's house, Cody refused to take his medication. After Liz explained that it was not optional, he threw his pills and screamed, "Dad said I shouldn't be taking all of this stuff, anyway."

Cody tore through the house furiously filling his backpack. "That's it! I'm done here!"

When he tucked his toy gun into one of the side pockets, Liz's stomach dropped.

"You are *not* leaving this house!" she insisted as she stood in the doorway in an attempt to block him. Cody pushed through, escaped into the backyard, and disappeared into the darkness.

With a recent news story fresh in her mind of a child who was shot by an officer for pointing a toy gun, Liz had no choice but to call 911.[5] She did not want Cody killed by mistake.

"I need help," she cried. "My son just left with a black backpack and is wearing dark clothing. He isn't in his right mind. It's a long story, but we think he has this condition called PANDAS. He has a toy gun with him—a *toy* gun—and I want to make sure you guys know that it is *not* real, so you do *not* shoot him by accident."

By the time the officers got to her house, Liz was beside herself. They told her that for them to help, she had to sign a petition charging Cody with running away.

The only thing she cared about at that moment was keeping Cody alive and safe, which meant it would be best if they kept him overnight. But to do so, Liz also had to sign a petition against her son for assault. Cody had shoved her aside to get out the back door. She would not call this an assault, but it was the only way they would keep him.

In desperation, she followed their instructions. She had seen first-hand that none of her tools were strong enough to combat ODD.

---

5   **A note from the author:** You might be wondering why I'd call the cops again after vowing that I wouldn't ever let Cody go back to the detention center. Trying to force him to take his meds—the only thing I knew that could lessen the behaviors of a flare—caused this explosion. I knew psych meds hadn't worked in the past, but I thought maybe we hadn't given them enough of a chance. I was willing to try anything at this point. I was rethinking everything I thought I had decided on. You might be familiar with ODD, but I had never seen it in my son... until this time. Despite how strongly I felt about Cody going back to the detention center, I was willing to allow that if it meant my son would be spared his life. I did *not* want him to be mistaken for a criminal and be shot!

MORE IN-HOME DETENTION

Within the week, Liz and John were summoned to a Department of Children's Services emergency family meeting at the detention center. Cody was allowed out of his cell to attend the meeting.

With a team gathered for Cody's welfare, Liz felt hopeful. *Maybe you have to get a certain level to get the team of professionals. Whatever it took! Finally, someone is going to help us.*

Ms. Ledford, the court-appointed guardian *ad litem*, called the meeting to order. After introductions were made, the discussions began.

"I need a court order for Cody to get an anti-DNase B titer test," Liz explained. She and John went on to tell the group about the behavioral problems at school and the presumed association with strep.

At the conclusion of the meeting, Liz was presented with more papers. These included some notes and a list of additional assignments Liz was mandated to complete along with all the other rules she had to follow for in-home detention, including getting family therapy, more therapy for Cody, and a case review by Vanderbilt Center of Excellence.

Cody had already had plenty of therapy. How would dragging everyone to family therapy help Cody's illness? Going to Vanderbilt to meet with a group of doctors, however, sounds like a great idea.

As Liz pushed through the double doors leading to the parking lot, she zeroed in on the notes and saw "Cody needs a tiger test."

Dear God! We are going backward. They don't even understand what test he needs. I'll just focus on the doctors.

Liz would have to use ferocity as the first corner piece in this puzzle—at least until she could find more pieces.

CHAPTER 6

Patient Dismissal

REST IN PEACE, RUSTY

Liz was up most of the night sorting through records she felt may be helpful for the doctors to review at their upcoming meeting. After a few hours of sleep, she was ready to dive back in, but as she passed by the front door, she noticed something unusual through the glass panel. Instead of waiting at the door like he always did, Rusty lay on the porch, not moving.

Liz opened the door, but Rusty still did not move. Their beloved pet of five years was dead.

He had been lethargic earlier that week, including when she let him out that morning. She felt terrible for not having taken him to the vet.

At dusk, everyone gathered around the sweet little grave Cody and Mark—the "manny"—made. Although Cody was devastated, Liz was grateful that he had been home from the detention center so he could enjoy Rusty's last days.

A NEW DIAGNOSTIC TEST

Dr. Meneely had consistently refused to order the titer test to see if Cody's body had elevated strep antibodies.

Maybe I'm asking for the wrong test. Perhaps I should be asking for something different.

Liz looked to see if there's a different test and was thrilled to learn that a new diagnostic test for PANDAS had become available. It was called the Cunningham Panel. She called Dr. Meneely's office right away.

"There's a new diagnostic test for PANDAS called the Cunningham Panel. This should help us finally know for sure if Cody has it," she explained to the nurse. Liz went on to explain that their housekeeper had a documented case of strep, and Cody had been exposed.

"Almost immediately, Cody became incredibly defiant and aggressive. Could you please ask Dr. Meneely to order the panel? I will pay for it out of pocket."

FIRED FOR PURSUING THE POSSIBILITY OF PANDAS

Instead of a return phone call, Liz received a letter from their pediatrician terminating his services. They would be allowed only acute care for the next thirty days while they found Cody a new primary care physician.

Dr. Meneely stated that Liz's ongoing non-compliance and disagreement with his medical advice to see a pediatric psychiatrist and/or neurologist was grounds for "patient dismissal."

He's firing us as his patients?! Is that even possible?

The letter continued: "Unfortunately, instead of accepting my medical advice for referrals, you prefer to pursue the possibility of PANDAS rather than dealing with Cody's behavioral problems.

It would be in Cody's best interest for you to follow up on the medical referrals that I have advised."

After numerous emails, phone calls, and conversations, how could he not have known that I have taken Cody to a child psychiatrist, thirty CBT sessions, put him on psych meds twice, implemented Total Transformation, and have done everything possible to get him an appointment with a pediatric neurologist? Plus, there were the guitar lessons, jujitsu, and wrestling.

Liz had gone above and beyond following Dr. Meneely's directions. She was simply requesting more than he was willing to consider.

The antibiotics and the tests that Dr. Meneely was denying us were the only things missing in the treatment plan. It would not have mattered what I had done because Dr. Meneely believed that all of Cody's problems were based on his behavioral choices.

Liz sent the pediatrician's office copies of the notes from each of the thirty CBT sessions via certified mail. She felt vindicated for proving that she had been compliant.

As if she did not have enough to deal with, though, Liz had no other option than to try and find Cody another pediatrician.

SOMETHING'S WRONG WITH MARK

Liz stacked a collection of binders, medical records, and selected research into Bankers Boxes, ready to head to a meeting at Vanderbilt's Center of Excellence regarding her son.

"John's coming to get Cody," she told Mark, "but I need you to watch the kids." As Mark heaved the last Bankers Box into the trunk, Liz noted that he was not looking so good. "Is everything okay?"

"I don't know. I've lost about thirty pounds," he admitted. "My family's getting worried."

"Please take care of yourself, Mark. I don't know where I'd find another maintenance manny!" She was not kidding.

As she drove to the hospital, Liz could not help but wonder why everyone in their household seems to be sick.

CASE REVIEW MEETING

Top-notch doctors from a prestigious university were attending Cody's case-review meeting, and Liz was eager to explain the situation to the group for their expert input. It was hard to get through the story without crying. Choking back tears, she ended with a plea: "He needs this test called the Cunningham Panel. Can any of you order it?"

"That has to be requested by Cody's doctor," one of the psychiatrists said.

Do I dare to explain that Cody's pediatrician has fired us? If we would prove he has PANDAS, Cody would get the treatment he needs, and he could get better. Wouldn't doing something about this situation be better than putting a child in jail? Aren't we all on the same team here?

The pediatrician spoke up, "Have you considered trying to get him into a clinical trial?"

Liz did not want to spend the time explaining how she had applied for two trials, but both applications had been rejected. Either the timing was not right, or Cody did not have the exact symptoms they were looking for. "I'll look into it again," she said. "But something needs to be done. I do not want Cody going back to juvenile jail."

"Well, if anything else happens," the psychiatrist suggested, "you should consider bringing him to Vanderbilt Psychiatry."

YET ANOTHER LIST

At the end of the meeting, Liz was given another useless to-do list instead of an order for the Cunningham Panel. She decided to draft her own, more proactive list.

One priority was to get her hands on Cody's full legal medical record—something she had learned about at the meeting. Liz had not heard that term before but as she looked further, it turned out you can request this from every provider. Strategically, Liz contacted every doctor and hospital who had ever called Cody a patient. The records came pouring in and once compiled, it was 800 pages—the perfect illustration of the magnitude of the task ahead.

Liz stared at the stack of papers as if it were in a foreign language, reminding herself: *You eat an elephant one bite at a time.* She put them in a huge, three-ring binder and committed to spending a little time each day digesting it.

She decided to reach out to Dr. Asher again. It had been three years since Liz had sat in her psychiatrist's office explaining Cody's medical mysteries.

Liz knew Dr. Asher was going out on a limb for them trying to help until they could find another doctor. She explained to her what the Cunningham Panel was and why she was adamant that Cody needed it to be done.

"I'm so sorry to even have to ask, but could you *please* order the panel? I'm embarrassed to say that Dr. Meneely fired us when I asked him for it, and the courts are no help at all. I don't know what else to do. I took him to my doctor who also sees children, but she doesn't know anything about PANDAS. Fortunately, she did know enough to give him some antibiotics for the boil he got after leaving the detention center. I'm at a complete loss," she explained.

"I've never seen anyone have to fight this hard to get a test done," Dr. Asher encouraged Liz. "Sure, I'll order it."

They had Cody's blood drawn and sent to Moleculera Labs.

For a change, Liz felt victorious. A single *yes* among the hundreds of *noes* was enough to renew her resolve.

CHAPTER 7

Up and Down

A MASSIVE EXPLOSION

The children had gone to spend a Friday night with their dad. When they came home the next morning, Michelle immediately went into her room and closed her door. Next followed Cody who seemed particularly out of sorts.

"Son, what's the matter?" Liz wanted to know.

"I got into a fight last night with two football players from another school—"

"What?! Where?!" Liz shouted.

"Downtown Franklin."

"Cody, you know you weren't even supposed to be there—now there's been a fight, and if any of this gets back to the courts, you'll be in serious trouble. And, what's more, they are going to blame *me*, not your dad! I can't believe this is happening."

Why won't he understand the consequences of an in-home detention violation?!

"Mom, can Caden spend the night?" Adam interrupted.

"That's fine, Adam," she agreed before Cody finished saying that one of the boys had tried to kick him in the head.

Cody was determined to get revenge and spent the better part of the day stewing. No matter how hard Liz tried to talk him out of taking revenge, he would not hear of it. She was worried about him, but he was safe at home, and life had to go on.

Later that night, Adam burst into her office. "Mom! Cody broke Caden's laptop in half and threw the theater seats across the room!"

Liz flung back her office chair. She dashed to the basement, adrenaline pumping. Cody was chasing after her, demanding to know what his mother was going to do. Liz wished there was an answer to that question.

Deep breath in.

She tried to remain calm, doing one thing at a time.

I'll move the music equipment upstairs while I try to figure this out.

"Give that back!" Cody grabbed the base of the microphone stand.

"Cody, no!" Liz held onto the stand.

As Cody let go, he hit his hand on the banister. When he saw a small cut, he shouted, "See, look what you've done! I'm calling the cops!"

Assuming it was an empty threat, Liz continued moving the equipment until she overheard Cody saying, "We need some help over here. Things are getting out of control."

He must have realized it was not a good idea, though, and quickly added: "Never mind. Nobody needs to come."

It was too late. The police were at their door within fifteen minutes. "You are *not* taking Cody to the detention center!" Liz insisted. "I did *not* call you, and I do *not* need your help."

But then Liz remembered what one of the doctors from the Vanderbilt Centers of Excellence had said just a few days ago: "If anything else happens, you should consider bringing him to Vanderbilt Psychiatry."

At least he won't be in the detention center.

They were going to take him one way or another, so Liz offered this as an alternate solution. The officers were sympathetic and changed the call to one of a medical nature. The younger officer noticed the music equipment, picked up a guitar, and started playing. This helped Cody calm down and open up to the officers. Cody explained that Adam had left the last cheeseburger out rather than putting it into the refrigerator, which had set him off.

Fortunately, the situation with the police was resolved amicably. Nevertheless, Cody was kindly escorted to an ambulance waiting outside the home and transported to Vanderbilt, Liz following closely behind.

"Is he homicidal or suicidal?" the nurse at Vanderbilt Hospital's emergency room asked. Not in his right mind, Cody spoke freely of his plans to get back at the two boys he had fought the night before, so technically, they had grounds to admit him to Vanderbilt Psychiatry.

Dr. Meneely said we could get it at Vanderbilt, so here we are.

MEDICAL TREATMENTS FOR PSYCHIATRIC SYMPTOMS

Liz soon realized that the psych hospital is no place for a child. She requested that her son be transferred to Vanderbilt Children's Hospital—after all, Cody's condition had improved when he was admitted there in the past.

Though Cody's attending psychiatrist agreed to order the anti-DNase B titer test, she would not agree to a transfer. Perhaps she thought Liz would let it go, but finally, she put in the order for an anti-DNase B titer test.

"Cody's titers are normal, Ms. Harris," the psychiatrist assured her, though unwilling to share the actual results.

Liz wanted to see the results for herself. She returned late that night and casually approached the front desk nurse. "Hey, can you pull up my son's labs and check something for me?"

Cody's results were 484 and were marked as critically high.

Why would she lie about something like that?

After ten days at the psychiatric hospital, Cody was given the green light to go home.

It was time for the discharge meeting and Liz stayed calm. "Can you prescribe him more antibiotics, please? As you are aware, he's been on Bactrim the entire time he has been here."

She was tentative as she continued. "I realize Bactrim isn't used for the kind of strep associated with PANDAS, but it seems to be helping both the boil *and* Cody's behavior. He took the last of the Bactrim yesterday, though. Can we please have more just in case that is, in fact, what is helping?"

"He's better because we changed his ADHD medication and added Luvox for the OCD," said the psychiatrist as if the problem had been solved.

Everyone works puzzles differently, but Liz had an advantage with the one before them. She had been working on this one from day one. She had watched as doctors switched her son from one kind of psych medication to another.

It hadn't worked before, and it wouldn't work now. What has worked so far was to start him on Bactrim.

Liz did not understand why Bactrim was helping. All she knew was what she saw with her own eyes. She witnessed Cody being exposed to strep via the housekeeper and, as a result, the last four weeks had been the next level of hell. And when her doctor put him on Bactrim to treat a boil, his behavior normalized.

The team at Vanderbilt Psychiatry clearly did not agree. Liz did not appreciate their closed-mindedness one bit. There was no sense trying to kick down a locked door, but she let them have a piece of her mind. "If you're set on looking at this from a psychological angle, how is it that you don't even know that his dog died recently?"

There was no stopping her. "I doubt that caused him to hurl theater chairs across a room, but I would say that qualifies as a loss for a child, and you seem obsessed with trauma and losses. Every time I ask for a plausible explanation for his behavior other than PANDAS, you insist it's stress from getting new siblings and from the divorce!"

Liz was livid. "I know plenty of people who have adopted children and have gotten divorced, and their kids don't end up in the psych ward! Stress can't be the answer to everything! I am stating for whatever legal medical record we are on right now, that *you* are the ones who have refused my son the *proper* medical treatment. And you outright lied about his titers! Why would you do that?"

Cody's psychiatrist went into character. "We didn't *lie* about the titers, Ms. Harris," she explained. "You may recall that they were 1,480 in 2010, so 484 is a *lot* lower. Some children simply have high titers. It shows that they had an infection in the past. If we go by the numbers, Cody doesn't have any current medical problems."

Cody doesn't have medical problems?! You've got to be kidding me. He has them. If only you'd be willing to turn this puzzle piece over and look at it!

Despite what the psychiatrists believed, Liz had seen that **the higher that number, the worse Cody was**.

It was no surprise then that Cody's behavior got worse within days of not having antibiotics. Liz knew antibiotics appeared to be the answer—not psych meds. But that was what the doctors insisted on giving him. She was more determined than ever to find a doctor who could continue his medical treatment, and with Cody away for ten days, she had had plenty of time to look into PANDAS treatment. While antibiotics did help, she had seen first-hand, how hard it was to get them.

There has to be another way.

AN APPOINTMENT TO SEE THE TOP PANDAS SPECIALIST

Liz was thrilled to share some good news with Cody for a change. "I've scheduled an appointment with the nation's top PANDAS specialist," she told Cody. "Dr. Latimer is the only doctor in the country who can give you IVIG[6] right in her office."

While it was still four months till that appointment, Liz was hopeful that once Dr. Latimer saw Cody, they could start the road to recovery.

From Liz's research, IVIG had recently been found to help children with PANDAS. Liz had no idea how she would pay for this expensive treatment other than hoping that Dr. Latimer would somehow be able to justify it to the insurance company.

---

6   Intravenous immunoglobulin (IVIG) is a treatment in which immunoglobins (antibodies) from the plasma of healthy donors are infused into a patient with autoimmune disorders. It can be helpful for patients who have autoimmune disorders.

RESULTS FROM THE CUNNINGHAM PANEL

The prospect of seeing a PANDAS specialist was not the only good news. Dr. Asher sent Liz the results from Cody's Cunningham Panel, **finally confirming that he indeed had PANS/PANDAS.**[7]

PANS? What is PANS?

Liz tried to digest the notion of this other similar-sounding condition. From what she could tell, it meant that kids with PANS flared when they were exposed to almost *any* infectious trigger, not just strep.

Please, God, don't let him have that. Having flares due to strep is hard enough.

To keep herself from curling up in a fetal position and giving up, Liz tried to convince herself that her son did not have PANS.

For once, PANDAS seemed manageable. Cody would be fine once they could get the strep out of his system and prevent him from getting it again.

This piece she had just been handed? Liz prayed it would not fit into Cody's puzzle.

BACK TO COURT

With the court hearings regarding the "runaway and assault" incident scheduled for the next day, Liz felt hopeful.

Now that Liz had test results in hand, she was convinced that Melinda Ledford, Cody's guardian *ad litem*, would help by providing referrals to doctors who knew how to treat this syndrome.

---

7   As a reminder, PANDAS is pediatric autoimmune neuropsychiatric disorders associated with streptococcal infections. PANS is pediatric acute-onset neuropsychiatric syndrome. More recently, PANDAS has been described as a subset of PANS.

To Liz's dismay, Ms. Ledford reported in court the next day that she had thoroughly investigated Cody's situation and found "absolutely no evidence of abuse or neglect. What I *did* find was a family who's really struggling."

Wait, what? They were looking for abuse or neglect?

With that, the judge dismissed Ms. Ledford from the case. The court-appointed—now court-dismissed—guardian simply closed her binder and left. Liz's hopes were shattered.

What about the "really struggling" family?

LOOKING FOR A NEW PEDIATRICIAN

After shaking off the disappointment that the courts would be not able to help them, Liz started her search for a new pediatrician. After making several more dead-end calls, Liz turned to Mission Clinic. Michelle and Adam's pediatrician, Dr. Brunner, agreed to try and help with Cody's PANDAS.

Relieved, Liz made the first available appointment—two months out!

The thought of having Cody thrown back in jail during a flare kept a fire lit under her, so Liz swallowed her pride and called Susan, Dr. Meneely's nurse to see if there was anything that could be done in the meantime.

"Listen, your letter said that you guys would still see Cody for acute care. We're still in the specified thirty-day window. I have test results to confirm that Cody has PANDAS, and he really needs to see a doctor."

Susan was kind enough to make Cody an appointment for later that week. "I'll book you with Dr. Brooks," she said.

That name sounded familiar to Liz. She flipped through the three-inch binder which she had been slowly digesting that contained all of Cody's legal medical records.

That's him! When Cody had his acute onset of OCD and I called their office, Dr. Brooks was the one who told us it might be PANDAS! He's the one who told us to go to Vanderbilt's emergency room!

A PANDAS PROTOCOL

Susan ushered them down a hallway Liz had never seen before. She handed the results of the Cunningham Panel to Dr. Brooks, and within a few minutes, a nurse did a rapid strep test and drew blood.

"Can you give Cody antibiotics to last until his appointment at Mission Clinic?" Liz asked. Before he had a chance to answer, she added, "And did you do the anti-DNase B test?"

"Yes, the protocol for children with suspected PANDAS is to draw blood, and if the results come back positive, to prescribe antibiotics," he explained.

Despite the rapid strep test being negative, Cody's anti-DNase B titers had risen to 584 within ten days, which was just cause for treatment. Dr. Brooks started Cody on Keflex, an antibiotic for strep.

The reality of what Dr. Brooks said sank in, and Liz could barely breathe.

There is a PANDAS protocol after all! At any point over the past three years, if Dr. Meneely had simply followed protocol, we would have been spared the heartache, the trouble at school, and the drama of juvenile detention and courts!

Feelings of frustration, grief, and hurt overtook her. Liz buried her head in her hands and cried.

CHAPTER 8

Little Boxes

WAY BEYOND OCD

The antibiotics Dr. Brooks prescribed seemed to be working. Gradually yet steadily, Cody began to improve. Wanting to make sure she was not missing something, Liz asked Mark if one of Cody's most tangible symptoms were improving.

"Mark, have you discovered any more of those little wooden boxes anywhere?" she asked. Cody had been hiding boxes all over the house that spring, and each one that Mark found had exactly the same items neatly placed inside.

He is hoarding but in a very unusual way.

"Now that you mention it, I haven't," Mark answered. "But have you looked in your garage lately? You may want to."

Liz went to the garage where she found Cody sitting in a "lab" he had fashioned—complete with a desk and a microscope he had found in a closet. On the cabinet were at least twenty little jars with samples of things like spiders, bugs, and dirt.

"I took samples from the yard of everything I could think of. I'm going to analyze them," Cody explained.

"Analyze them for what?"

"Whatever I have!" Cody answered confidently.

He seems to want to figure out this puzzle as much as I do. But the way he has this all organized? This is way beyond OCD.

WARNING SIGNS OF THINGS TO COME

Cody's symptoms were manageable, so when a family member called and offered Liz a weekend timeshare in New Orleans, she gladly accepted. Liz desperately needed a break after years of one crisis after another.

Liz invited Andrea to go along. She and Andrea had been friends for nearly twenty years, and when in New Orleans, they had just as much fun—if not more—than back when they were young. Monday morning rolled around too soon.

Andrea woke up with what seemed like a migraine. "You probably just had too much wine," Liz teased her friend. "You can sleep it off. I'll drive."

Andrea slept the whole way home. By the time they arrived back in Nashville, Andrea was not feeling any better. She was not able to make the two-hour drive home.

"How about you rest a little longer in the guest bedroom?" she offered.

When Andrea emerged several hours later looking and feeling even worse, Liz realized her friend was not hungover, she was sick.

We cannot expose Cody to anything!

Cody had greeted them at the door upon their return. Naturally, Andrea had hugged him before she laid down to rest.

"Does your throat hurt?" Liz asked nervously.

"No, I just feel weak and shaky."

Andrea doesn't have strep. We are going to be fine.

To be safe, Andrea self-isolated in the guest room.

Cody is still on the Keflex Dr. Brooks had given him. We are going to be fine.

Liz caught herself saying those words to herself over and over, hoping they were true.

Andrea stayed in isolation, and Cody stayed far away from her helping Mark build a new deck in the backyard.

By Tuesday night, Cody was blinking relentlessly.

"Mom," he complained, "my eyes are burning."

AN ONSLAUGHT OF TERRIBLE BEHAVIORS

Cody's behavior escalated within a week. Despite never having been taught to drive a car—much less a stick shift—he took Mark's car and ended up being arrested.

He had driven more than an hour to visit a girl he had met in the psych hospital, no less. He made it one mile from the house before he was pulled over.

When the police found some of his medications with him that he had recently been hoarding in wooden boxes again, so on top of everything else, they suspected he was dealing drugs.

The thirteen-year-old was sent back to the detention center.

By now, Liz had seen the pattern. When Cody was exposed to strep, he had a flare. But as far as she knew, Andrea did *not* have strep.

Despite being on an antibiotic for strep, Cody was in a full-blown flare. The reality began to sink in: Andrea must have a virus. If a virus caused Cody's flare, it would mean his PANDAS could be PANS.

No! God, please, no!

They had an appointment scheduled with Dr. Latimer—the PANDAS specialist—but that was still three months away.

I cannot believe we've even made it this far. How are we going to make it till then?

Cody exhibited an onslaught of abhorrent behaviors and horrible decisions, as if he had lost all executive functioning, having no ability to make decisions of his own.

This was far beyond simply bad behavior—it was as if he did not know he was doing anything wrong. His behavioral changes had more ups and downs than the Rocky Mountains!

GETTING AN ELECTRONIC ANKLE MONITOR

Liz was determined to get Cody home from the detention center and safely confined—*any* way possible. "I have researched electronic ankle monitoring companies," she told the judge, handing him a flyer with the information, "and I would like to request that Cody wear one from *this* company."

Liz never imagined herself being in this position, but there she was, working out a deal with a judge for Cody to wear an ankle monitor rather than to be locked up.

The judge ordered that Cody wear an ankle monitor provided by the court and warned her, "Ms. Harris, if you cannot take care of your child, the state will take control of him."

Disillusioned and feeling like the state had no intention of helping anyone, Liz left the courthouse in tears.

OUT OF CONTROL

Either the GPS on the ankle monitor was not working, or the lone woman at the response center tasked with following the movements of clients was either sleeping through the alarms, or she was paying no attention. Whatever the reason, it did not take long for Cody to discover that the monitoring service was not working.

As a result, Liz and Mark spending endless hours trying to keep Cody from scrambling out of windows.

Cody also figured out how to order goods online using his mom's debit card. She would hide her wallet, but before she knew it, purchases would show up on the doorstep again for goods no thirteen-year-old could walk into a store and buy.

Liz yet again called her bank to get a new card. "How is it possible that he knows how to do all this?" she vented to Mark. It's like Cody has access to a part of his brain that no human should have. How is it possible that he knows how to do all this? He's *never* been exposed to behaviors like this."

This behavior came about practically overnight, so Liz googled what part of the brain is responsible for criminal activity, convinced that something has to be wrong with that spot in his brain.

Is it the frontal lobe? The amygdala? Looks like it could be either.

Liz knew little about the different brain region's impact on behavior, but she found it surprisingly reassuring that there was medical literature making the connection between behavioral issues and brain damage of some sort.

To make things even worse, Cody barely slept, giving him even more time to act out his compulsions. This meant Liz had to stay up for long stretches to keep an eye on Cody who was completely out of control.

It seemed almost impossible to keep Cody safe until they would finally see Dr. Latimer, the PANDAS specialist.

SEEING DR. BENDER AT MISSION CLINIC

Though Cody had displayed no traditional symptoms of a viral infection, his behavior was dire. To get the root of the flare, Liz needed confirmation that Cody had indeed contracted a virus.

The only upside to his latest flare was that it coincided with Cody's first appointment with Dr. Brunner, the pediatrician at Mission Clinic—the appointment they had scheduled two months prior.

"Cody's ears are ringing and hurting," Liz explained.

Dr. Brunner examined Cody and confirmed that he seemed to have an ear infection. "The problem isn't only in your ear," he told Cody. "You have an acute upper-respiratory virus."

He turned to Liz. "Since Cody's already on an antibiotic, there's nothing we can do until it runs its course."

Liz just sat there, staring blankly.

Run its course?! Do you even know what that means? **Cody indeed seemed to have PANS.** *Most mothers hear sneezing and sniffling when their child is sick. Oh, to be that fortunate. When my son is sick, I hear sirens. I hear the squawk of police walkie-talkies and the slam of a jail-cell door.*

This must stop!

THIS TIME, CODY'S DAD CALLED 911

Mark came to Liz with the news that Karen, his girlfriend, was pregnant. Mark asked if she could move in with him in the lower level.

While she was uncomfortable with the arrangement, the house was big enough, so Liz agreed to let Karen move in. She could not risk Mark leaving at a time like this. Cody had to stay safe until Liz could get him to Dr. Latimer. It was truly her last hope.

They made it through two weeks, and it was only two days before leaving to see Dr. Latimer in Maryland when Cody's behaviors started getting out of control. He pushed Liz and Mark to their limits.

Liz was doing everything possible to respect the court's order. But when she tried to take Cody's video games, he exploded. Mark was not feeling well and Liz needed backup, so she called John for help, describing Cody's behavior when she took video games away from him.[8]

"This is insane, John!" she exclaimed. "The juvenile courts are putting both of our lives at risk."

Alarmed, John called 911.

To Liz's horror, emergency vehicles swarmed her home yet again, and the police made their way to Cody's room. Liz pushed her way past the officers who blocked his doorway. When she saw a red laser pointed at her son's chest, she fell to her knees.

"Don't hurt him!" she screamed. "He is sick!"

Cody stood frozen. The irises of his eyes were not showing at all; his pupils completely dilated.

Instead of sending him to juvenile detention, the police allowed Liz to take Cody to the Vanderbilt emergency room. But with the fear that they may keep him for ten days causing them to miss the appointment with Dr. Latimer, Liz took him back home.

Liz resumed the round-the-clock guard duty.

---

8   **A note from the author:** As crazy as it seems, the in-home detention mandate forbade the use of any electronics. This was nothing other than cruel since playing video games on occasion was the only thing that tended to keep Cody calm.

GOING TO SEE THE PANDAS SPECIALIST (AT LAST!)

The last thing Liz wanted to do was to go on a road trip with an out-of-control teenager. But missing their appointment with Dr. Latimer was not an option.

Protecting Cody was exhausting, but the prospect of possibly finding some answers kept Liz alert. Little did she know how challenging it would be to get to Dr. Latimer's office in one piece.

On the way to Maryland to see Dr. Latimer, a magnificent rainbow stretched through the pale sky with a streak of the most vibrant colors Liz had ever seen. It gave her hope.

"Cody, that is God's promise to us," she smiled. "We're on the right track. Once you get this IVIG, you'll be a lot better. Those flares should be gone forever."

She desperately hoped that the newest research would prove to be true.

Cody seemed calm, like he often did during the day. But like other days during a flare, something shifted mid-afternoon. That day was no different. By the evening, it was like Cody had changed into a different person.

Liz knew that if they could get through the night, the morning would bring hope. Knowing that Cody's ankle monitor was useless, Liz had to stay up to make sure he stayed put. But she was physically and emotionally drained and had to stop halfway there to sleep for the night.

Once they were checked in, she tried to stay awake until Cody fell asleep but to no avail. No matter how hard she tried, though, she fell asleep. When she woke up and Cody was in the bed next to her, it seemed like a miracle.

They stopped for some breakfast before setting off again.

ACTING ON COMPULSIONS

"Mom, I have to tell you something," Cody said during the next leg of their trip. "I got out of the hotel last night."

Liz's heart dropped.

Why would he readily admit that? It just didn't make sense.

She was not happy that he had escaped but felt that it was a good sign that he confessed. Cody's choices did not seem like they were his at all—they seemed more like a compulsion—ones that he wanted to stop rather than hide.

Liz contacted the monitoring company, asking them to set a new perimeter around their hotel in Maryland. Feeling confident in her management of the situation, Liz slid under the covers and fell asleep with the car keys tucked safely under her pillow.

Within an hour, something woke her up.

Where's Cody?

Liz bolted upright. Grabbing her robe, she darted down the hallways of the hotel before pushing open the front doors. Her car was gone.

Liz raced back to her room and called the monitoring company. "What in the hell are you doing?" she screamed at the operator. "Cody's gone! He is a thirteen-year-old boy, driving around an area close to Washington, D.C. with *your* ankle monitoring device on! You have only *one* job and that is to monitor my son and call me if he leaves the perimeter we had set!"

Liz was not only furious at the operator; she was frantic with concern for her son.

The operator offered to try to get Cody back to the hotel through the audio on his GPS device. By the time Cody pulled back into the hotel parking lot, the SUV was dented, but Cody was safe.

After recovering from the shock, Liz asked the front desk for a cot. She pushed it against the door and slept there, successfully preventing Cody from slipping out again.

MEETING OTHER KIDS WITH PANDAS

Sitting in the waiting room was an enlightening and educational experience. It gave the moms of kids with PANDAS a chance to swap horror stories. One mother told of how her son would throw himself into oncoming traffic during a flare. Liz was dumbfounded.

What in the world is wrong with these children? I don't remember hearing about anything like this when I was growing up. These children seem to be possessed! They are either compelled to kill themselves or to kill others. This can't be happening.

Hearing stories from other moms in person freaked Liz out.

Cody, on the other hand, seemed to be relieved to see other kids who were like him. He leaned over and whispered, "Mom, these kids are like me."

Cody was older than the other patients, but they seemed just as sick as he was. Perhaps it should have made Liz feel better, but it only made her angrier that a solution had not been found for their children.

That there was a doctor's office full of kids like this with a many-month-long waiting list made her shiver.

MEETING DR. LATIMER

When it was their turn, Liz walked into the doctor's office and resolutely set the Bankers Box full of records and research in the middle of her desk. Looking her in the eyes, her greeting was more like a plea for survival. "I sure hope you can help my child."

After reviewing the medical records and completing a thorough evaluation to the tune of $900—no insurance accepted—Dr. Latimer set her pen down, looked at Liz, and said, "It *is* PANDAS."[9]

Liz did not ask about the possibility of it being PANS, but she did learn that the "stealing" Cody had been doing—his backpack was full of medical supplies he had managed to acquire while changing for his evaluation—was simply hoarding. For the time being, she felt vindicated.

The country's leading PANDAS expert has officially diagnosed Cody once and for all!

Being certain of what you are dealing with is the first step toward a solution.

After two days of IVIG treatments and IV-administered steroids for the brain inflammation, Dr. Latimer comforted Liz that she would start seeing improvements in about six weeks, at which time Dr. Latimer wanted to see Cody again.

She encouraged Liz to slowly wean him from the psych meds. "His symptoms will go away in the order in which they came." Liz had barely processed the phrase, *six weeks* when Dr. Latimer slowed down, looked Liz in the eyes, and continued, "And Ms. Harris, you'll need to know that Cody will get worse before he gets better."

How is that possible? How can he get even worse?

Still numb with terror, Liz stopped at the front desk to book the follow-up appointment and to write the check for $18,000.

---

9   PANDAS is a clinical diagnosis based on a thorough review of health history. It is usually supported with testing, but finding a doctor who knows which tests, how to interpret those tests, and put together the correct treatment plan is an overwhelming obstacle for most families.

Having depleted her cash reserves to keep everything afloat thus far, she had to humble herself and ask a family member for help. Fiercely independent as she was, having to ask family for financial help was a difficult step. But Liz was convinced that once she filed a grievance with the insurance company, she would be able to repay the money as well as pay for any future treatment.

Liz also knew that if she could push the treatment through insurance, it would open the door for treatment for other families too.

Cody seemed more like his old self as they started their journey home. But Liz had a heaviness to her.

"What's wrong, Mom?" he asked as they got back on the interstate.

How can I tell my son—who believes he's cured—that he is going to get worse?

Wanting to avoid another scene at a hotel, Liz drove home without more than a short break or two. They pulled up at home fifteen hours later, bone tired.

CALLING FOR HELP

Dr. Latimer was right: Cody was worse the next day. He could not sit still, and he paced around the house nonstop.

Liz was exhausted; she needed backup. Mark was not doing well—he was suffering from ever-worsening headaches—so she called Andrea.

"Thanks for coming," Liz greeted her at the door.

"No problem." Andrea set her bags down.

Liz had been awake for thirty-six hours, so she simply said, "That ankle monitor doesn't work, so you *have* to stay on him like white on rice." With that, she headed to bed and fell into a deep sleep.

The next thing Liz knew, it was three in the morning, and someone was banging on the door. It was an officer who explained that there had been an accident.

Liz noticed that her car was gone. "Is Cody all right?" Her heart was pounding.

"Yes, he's fine. He's been taken to the Williamson County Detention Center. But your car has been totaled."

Liz learned that Cody had escaped five times that night to see friends across the street before he finally wrecked the car.

Andrea was beside herself. "I was checking on him every thirty minutes!"

"I believe you," Liz assured her friend. "But he can slip out and slip back in ten."

BACK IN THE DETENTION CENTER

The only option was to get Cody into a treatment facility. Finding a facility equipped to handle Cody's complex medical needs while also managing his psych symptoms was next to impossible. The controversy with diagnosis codes made things that much more difficult.

I have to find him someplace to go other than jail... Cody's supposed to be experiencing recovery, *not* punishment!

Liz's mom, Carol—a counselor at NeuroRestorative, a brain rehabilitation facility—offered a possible solution. Her company had an adolescent center for brain rehab in Illinois. "If we can get him into that program, it would be better for Cody's recovery than a jail cell," she suggested.

Liz could not agree more. She began the application right away. Once she learned that Cody's insurance benefits would cover the stay, she scheduled the clinical interview.

APPEARING BEFORE A NEW JUDGE

Cody's detention hearing for his most recent slew of charges included two in-home detention violations, a curfew violation, driving without a license, and failing to report an accident.

Liz set aside the criminal issues to focus on the medical ones. Nothing could distract her from getting Cody where he needed to be, but this time, she was in front of a snarky Judge Guffee.

Cody's lawyer had to ask permission for Liz to take her son to the brain rehab center for an evaluation. The judge was not keen on the idea. She was more interested in making Liz look like a villain for letting Cody get out of the hotel room during their previous out-of-state appointment.

She eventually agreed, but they were not allowed to stay in a hotel room overnight. And if Cody were to be denied access to the program, Liz had to have him back to the juvenile detention center by nine the same night of the interview.

Determined to make the trip without incidents, Liz invited Carol to accompany them.

CHAPTER 9

Solitary Confinement

HEADING TO BRAIN REHAB

Cody had spent well over a week in a cell before the day of his clinical interview arrived. The first stop on Liz's road trip to Illinois was to pick her son up.

After an hour or so in the car, it became clear that something had shifted. Liz could not help but notice that Cody was more peaceful and less fidgety. When she looked into his eyes, she could almost recognize her son.

The next stop was her mother's home. "This isn't just wishful thinking," she told Carol. "The IVIG seems to be working."

The clinical interview was nerve-wracking, but it was worth every minute of the three hours it took. They were told they would be notified within hours whether or not Cody was accepted. Liz had no reason to believe Cody would be denied access.

Rightfully so.

Liz, Carol, and Cody were grabbing a bite to eat when she received an email with the good news.

"Congratulations on Cody's acceptance. On Monday, we will obtain a letter of medical necessity from Dr. Latimer and submit a treatment plan to the insurance company."

Liz was confused. Twice, Cody had been admitted at Vanderbilt Hospital without any delay, so she was not prepared for a delay. They would have to wait till Monday.

Should we drive back home? Or am I supposed to request permission to wait?

Carol assured Liz that waiting on insurance approval is standard procedure. She suggested Liz and Cody spend the weekend at her house. Cody had been accepted into the program, so technically, they were not going against Judge Guffee's orders.

This also afforded Carol time to teach Liz some strategies to calm Cody, ones Carol used with brain injury sufferers. Cody was slowly but surely improving. The techniques were working so well that Liz had felt comfortable in decreasing his psych meds as Dr. Latimer had recommended.

But Dr. Latimer was out of the office on Monday, so the letter of medical necessity and thus Cody's admittance into the program was delayed by another day. Or so Liz thought.

Not accepting the diagnosis code, the insurance company denied the claim. Liz appealed but was denied a second time.[10] The appeals took time, and by then, Liz and Cody had been at her mom's place for three weeks.

---

10 **A note from the author:** The insurance company rejected coverage of the treatment stating that although Dr. Latimer had signed a letter of medical necessity for brain rehabilitation at NeuroRestorative, she could not ethically place him in a facility she had no direct knowledge of. The only facility Dr. Latimer could legitimately recommend was Rodgers in Michigan, which had a waiting list of nearly a year. There was a consultant I could hire for $6,000 who could attempt to find placement for Cody, but there were no guarantees. It was not within my budget to take such a pricy risk.

TROUBLE WITH THE JUDGE

Once the judge learned that Cody had not yet been admitted, she called Liz demanding to know where Cody was.

Liz explained that he had been approved for the program but that their insurance details had caused a delay. "The rehab center will take TennCare, though. Is there any chance you could help us get approved for TennCare?"

The judge was seething. She did not care one bit how Cody was doing. Instead, she demanded that Cody be brought back to the detention center immediately.

Cody's attorney explained that the district attorney was considering extraditing Cody to the detention center. "The judge may charge you with contempt of court," the attorney warned Liz. "You may want to contact your lawyer."

Contempt of court for trying to get my child into a brain rehab center? Isn't that my job as a parent?

Cody was terrified during the ride back down to Tennessee. He begged his mother not to let them put him in solitary confinement as they had done before.

This was the first time Liz had heard mention of solitary confinement. Agonizing over what Cody was going through, she turned to look out the window so he could not see the tears streaming down her face. She had no idea what to do to protect her son.

PERMISSION TO SEE THE SPECIALIST: DENIED

When Liz dropped Cody off at the detention center, she tried to stay strong. She gave him a big hug before returning to her car where she broke down crying. She had to get Cody into a treatment center.

Merely three days after being back in the detention center, Liz learned he had been put in solitary confinement, the thing he feared most. Liz was in anguish. Her son was stuck in a 7' x 11' cell, and he was only allowed out if she came to do homework with him.

After calling everyone she could think of, it was suggested that she reach out to the Office of the Administrative Courts. Per their instructions, Liz called the Disability Law and Advocacy Center of Tennessee and lodged a complaint.

After two and a half weeks of dead ends, NeuroRestorative or any other facility capable of managing Cody's medical needs were not options. Cody's follow-up appointment with Dr. Latimer was three days away, but the warden made it clear that Cody would not be attending.

Why don't they want Cody to see Dr. Latimer?

"What? He has to go to that appointment. Dr. Latimer will have new recommendations now that the IVIG has been successful. He may not need a facility at all!" Liz insisted. "Can he at least go see Dr. Asher? Her office is right up the street?"

Although Liz had spent the last six months trying to get Cody from Dr. Asher, the psychiatrist, to Dr. Latimer, the neurologist, it now seemed as if anything was better than nothing.

"We can probably do that," the warden said as he walked away.

Liz left the detention center and went straight to her attorney.

"Maybe they just don't understand," was the only explanation he could come up with.

He helped her file a motion for an emergency hearing along with the requests the Cody be allowed to attend the appointment with Dr. Latimer, that he be moved out of solitary confinement, and the circumstances surrounding NeuroRestorative.

Despite having ample evidence of isolation having devastating long-term effects on juveniles, Judge Guffee ordered that Cody stay in solitary confinement where he was to remain for the weeks up until his final adjudication. She also issued an unwritten no-contact order. Cody was not allowed to speak to, nor receive visits from either of his parents.

The judge reappointed Melinda Ledford, the guardian *ad litem*, and issued an order for an expedited forensic psychological evaluation for a JCCO[11] to determine if Cody was competent to be adjudicated.

Cody's final hearing was set for two weeks out.

This puzzle is turning into a horror movie. Make it stop, please!

The next day Cody was transported to see Dr. Asher who reported that Cody's PANDAS symptoms had reduced from ten out of ten to zero out of ten. But the most telling was the handwriting samples before and after IVIG, which showed an astonishing improvement.

Cody slowly deteriorated as he sat alone, in that cold, dark cell for twenty-three hours a day isolated from anyone and everyone who loved him.

Up until now, Liz believed that the majority of Cody's psychiatric symptoms—if not all—were the result of a medical condition. But now, things had changed, and she would have to concede that the psychological torture he was enduring could indeed result in some of the same symptoms.

The day of Cody's final adjudication arrived, and Ms. Ledford had the result of Cody's JCCO evaluation. Dr. Asher's report was

---

11 A juvenile court commitment order (JCCO) is supposed to be used to determine if a juvenile qualified for involuntary commitment at a psychiatric facility. It is also used to determine if a juvenile is competent to understand the adjudication process—that is, if they'd be able to understand what is happening during a trial.

completely ignored and there was no mention of Dr. Latimer's recommendation for continued treatment at Rogers Memorial.

Liz asked to see the report, and Ms. Ledford sheepishly handed her the sixteen-page document. After seeing Liz flip straight to the recommendation on the last page, Ms. Ledford snatched it away. She explained that the report was confidential and was to be used to secure Cody's placement.

ADHD, OCD, ODD, and conduct disorder?! Continue his psychiatric medications and send him to a residential treatment center?!

Ms. Ledford went on to explain that they would only release Cody was if he were to temporarily live with John. John would be under court order to work with Ms. Ledford for placement. Liz reluctantly agreed.

Anything to get Cody out of that place.

Being careful not to tip off Ms. Ledford that she had overheard the name of the facility being considered, she sat quietly through the proceedings.

Once court was adjourned and Cody was leaving the courtroom with his father, Ms. Ledford walked over, "Ms. Harris, I need you to sign this," as she handed her the petition for dependency and neglect.

Liz was not going to sign anything else presented to her by anyone involved with this circus. "I want a hearing. I said Cody could temporarily stay with John. I will not sign a one-sided court document."

She turned to walk away with Ms. Ledford threatening that if she did not sign the document, things could get much worse.

Worse than this? I doubt that.

After arriving home, Liz gathered all the medical documentation she had and faxed it to the corporate headquarters for the facility Ms. Ledford had mentioned.

My son is not going to some godforsaken dungeon just to be further traumatized and forgotten about.

Liz had learned that it was illegal for a facility to accept a patient if they could not accommodate their medical needs. There was a substantial fine involved which Liz reminded them of when she called to confirm receipt of the records.

As Liz was faxing medical records, Ms. Ledford was busy faxing the new court order to Dr. Latimer, the insurance company, and Cody's school. It seemed as if Liz had just lost her rights to make medical decisions on Cody's behalf.

They want to make me look like I have Munchausen's by proxy as grounds for removing permanent custody so they can avoid the lawsuit I'm going to file.

Liz had seen it happen before on the PANDAS Facebook pages and now, it was happening to them.

TRYING TO PROTECT CODY

"Cody has an unmet medical need," Ms. Ledford had said. Though Liz knew that by *medical* she meant *psychiatric,* but she also knew that antibiotics and IVIG were the only things that had made Cody's situation manageable.

Liz needed to find a PANDAS doctor who could give him IVIG without the distractions of court proceedings and insurance. If she could find one, John could schedule the appointment and take Cody.

Liz discovered a PANDAS conference in Atlanta that weekend. She drove all night, racing to the sign-in table just before the first lecture started. All the speakers made some helpful points, but one speaker stood out—a certain Dr. Trifiletti, a man most referred to by his nickname, Dr. T.

One thing he said had stuck with her: "To treat PANDAS, you have to treat the infection."

What did he mean by that?

Dr. T also told them that he could control PANDAS *without* IVIG.

Did I hear right?

Despite the good response Cody had shown to IVIG treatment, the court order that robbed Liz of making medical decisions on Cody's behalf was cause for denial of her grievance.

Financially, additional IVIG treatment would be next to impossible.

Up to that point, Liz was not aware of an alternative treatment option. Finding someone who might be able to treat Cody without the expensive IVIG procedure felt godsent.

Liz's heart was set on Dr. T taking on Cody's case.

After his speech, Liz pushed through the crowd of other die-hard PANDAS mothers and handed Dr. T a few of Cody's labs.

"Please, you have to help my son," she said between tears. "I can't begin to describe all that PANDAS has done to our family, and now, I'm pretty sure it's progressed to PANS. Please, can you help?"

"Any mother who loves her son this much…" Dr. T said. "Sure, I will try to help him." The hope within Liz flickered brighter.

MICHELLE'S NOT FEELING WELL, EITHER

Meanwhile, Michelle mentioned several concerns including a heart issue, headaches, and difficulty sleeping. Liz took her to see her pediatrician at Mission Clinic.

"Hmm… you know, anxiety can cause these symptoms," Dr. Brunner observed. "Let's send her to one of the therapists here."

It was true that their lives were stressful, so Liz agreed to schedule Michelle for a psychological assessment. For the headaches, Dr. Brunner recommended that Michelle keep a headache journal so he could try to discern the cause.

"Adam's having issues as well," Liz explained. "The ADD medication isn't doing much, and I swear he would forget his head if it weren't attached to his body."

Dr. Brunner recommended that Adam get a psychological assessment as well.

"Can you put in a referral for Cody too?" Liz wanted Cody to process the trauma of five weeks in solitary confinement—and all that had gone with it—as soon as possible.

The court order forbade him from speaking of anything negative that happened while he was in the detention center, and Liz knew that the longer Cody was forced to keep quiet, the deeper the wounds could grow.

"We know he has been traumatized, and hopefully I will have him back in my custody by the time you can schedule his assessment," she explained.

"Sure," Dr. Brunner agreed.

FIGHTING A CORRUPT JUVENILE COURT

John called her later that day with big news. "You missed a lot in court this morning. Melinda Ledford nonsuited the petition against you."

"She what?"

Surely, I heard him wrong.

"Yeah, she dropped the whole thing!" John added, "I can drop Cody off to you this afternoon if that works for you."

"I get Cody back?" Liz was ecstatic. "Of course, it works for me!"

All it had taken was Connie Reguli, Esq. to depose Dr. Asher, Cody's former psychiatrist, and fight on Liz's behalf against a system that is at times much more than simply flawed. Liz was well aware that no other lawyer would have prevailed. But Connie was more than a fighter. She was insatiable when it came to the protection of children.

Liz scheduled a remote appointment with Dr. T to let him know the good news. Within the hour, Liz received an email with an extensive lab order.

Much relieved that Dr. T undoubtedly knew what to look for, Liz went to get Cody and took him straight to the lab for a blood draw.

Overwhelmed with gratitude, Liz and Cody enjoyed a nice dinner out that evening.

ELEVATED THYROID ANTIBODIES

The following week, the results of Cody's tests were in, and Liz scheduled a remote appointment with Dr. T to go over them. But not before she rushed over to Williamson Medical Center for her copy of the results.

It was the first time she had spoken with Dr. T since Cody's return home.

"We need to figure out what's going on with Cody's thyroid. His thyroid antibodies are very high, but his immune system looks fine," the specialist told her. "It could be Hashimoto's encephalopathy, though. We should look into that." Dr. T ordered additional testing.

Now his thyroid?

This was overwhelming. Liz needed more puzzle pieces. Some of the pieces she had been given so far simply were not fitting in anywhere.

She pored over the thirty-five pages of unfamiliar words and numbers on the new set of labs. It was all starting to look like Greek to her.

Liz decided to take a break and go over to the hospital to visit Mark and Karen's brand-new twins. Although Karen was deathly ill right before the delivery, she had successfully given birth to adorable twin boys.

To Liz's delight, Karen gave her the honor of naming them. Liz carefully chose the names Zachary and Hunter.

Maybe babies are just what we all needed—they sure lighten the mood!

GETTING ANTIVIRALS

A year before, when Liz was looking for a local PANDAS doctor, she found Dr. Karlton[12] on the PANDAS website. The first available appointment he had, though, was a year later. At the time, Liz scheduled it while continuing to pursue other options.

She had since met Dr. T and had her heart set on him treating Cody. But Liz had seen Dr. Karlton at the PANDAS conference in Atlanta where she had first heard Dr. T.

She hoped he might be willing to work with Dr. T to see Cody in case he had another flare.

After examining Cody and looking at a summary of his recent labs, Dr. Karlton concluded that Cody had viral triggers. "In fact," Dr. Karlton explained, "*any* infection could trigger Cody's behaviors."

"So, it's definitely PANS?"

---

12   Not his real name.

"Based on these labs, it sure looks like it. His HHV-6 is really high."[13]

That fit with what Liz had experienced and observed regarding Cody's various flare episodes. "Okay, so what can I do?"

He gave Cody a new prescription for antibiotics as well as an antiviral, adding, "Cody has major sensitivity, so in addition to treating the infection, we need to limit anything that could potentially cause inflammation or infection."

He scribbled a list of foods to avoid—including foods with food dyes, heavy metals, gluten, dairy, sugar, high-fructose corn syrup, preservatives, and MSG—as well as potential environmental triggers.

Tears welled up.

In addition to keeping him away from all possible infections, now he cannot eat gluten, dairy, or sugar, either? Cody won't be able to enjoy any of his favorite foods again!

Dr. Karlton also handed her an extensive list of supplements Cody should be taking and suggested that Liz continue working with doctors who could administer IVIG.

I have to find out what causes PANS/PANDAS! God, please let Dr. T be right. Please let there be a way other than IVIG. Please let there be a cure!

It all felt too much for Liz—like Dr. Karlton just spilled coffee all over the puzzle pieces Liz had meticulously turned over and had started to connect.

---

13   Human Herpesvirus 6 (HHV-6) is a set of two closely related herpes viruses known as HHV-6A and HHV-6B. HHV-6B infects nearly all human beings, typically before the age of three, and often results in fever, diarrhea, sometimes with a rash known as roseola. It is thought that once it runs its course, this infection typically lays dormant throughout life.

GETTING PHYSICALLY SICK

Within a few days, Cody became physically sick. He was stuffy and so lethargic that he could do nothing but sleep.

Maybe those antivirals are working so that he is getting physical symptoms of disease now rather than psychological symptoms. Maybe he's better already. One could hope…

Liz had no way of knowing that she was spot on with these observations.

Cody could barely get out of bed, so he stayed home from school for two weeks. But without a doctor's note, Liz was forced to put him back in school. Somehow, Cody made it through his finals.

THE DEATH OF A BABY

As soon as the twins were healthy enough, they came home. Mark and Karen had planned on moving to a place of their own once the babies were born. But the twins were struggling and were underweight. Hunter was also spitting up a lot and stayed dehydrated. He had to have surgery.

Liz agreed that the now-family-of-four could stay until the babies were well. After all, it was nice having new life in the house, and with the kids home for the summer, they loved playing with the babies. Liz enjoyed watching them when she could.

"I'm way too old to be having babies," Mark admitted to Liz. "I've been having the worst headaches lately. And last night, my side was hurting so badly, I drove myself to the emergency room. They're sending me to the gastroenterologist. I'll need some time off to go."

Mark left for his doctor's appointment and then went to visit his sister who lived nearby. Meanwhile, Karen took the boys and visited her family. Early the next morning, Mark texted Liz. "I won't be coming in for work today. Baby Zach died in his sleep last night."

Liz's heart sank. She immediately called Mark. "Please say it's not true! What happened?" As hard as it was to fathom, Zach had simply quit breathing sometime during the night.

"Wait. Didn't the babies get their shots last week?"

"Zachary got them, but Hunter was still too weak from the surgery a few weeks back, so he didn't," Mark explained. Karen said it was that pneumonia shot. They told her it would not cause SIDS, but she did not believe them.

Their world came to a halt. Liz bought an urn for baby Zach, and she and the children attended the funeral. Cody was devastated; he had bonded with the twins. Karen and Mark were heartbroken.

The next several weeks at the Harris home were full of sadness and tears.

Why does there seem to be something wrong with everyone around me?!

CHAPTER 10
Could This Mean Something?

FINDING A CORNER PIECE OF THE PUZZLE

A few weeks later, Cody had finished the medicine prescribed by Dr. Karlton. The results of the second set of labs ordered by Dr. T were not in yet, and his OCD and anxiety were coming back.

Had Cody caught something again? Was his IVIG wearing off, or did he need more antibiotics for the strep that may still be there?

According to Dr. T's initial tests, there was nothing wrong with Cody's immune system. It made no sense that someone with a perfectly functioning immune system would need more antibodies, anyway. Maybe more comprehensive tests needed to be run?

Fortunately, a few days later, the results from the additional testing were in and Liz scheduled a follow-up call with Dr. T.

In addition to the high thyroid antibodies, Cody's antibodies to streptococcal pneumonia[14] were through the roof. His labs also showed a *Mycoplasma pneumoniae* infection.[15]

The pneumococcal titer test results showed a response to the twenty-three strains tested. Liz was on overload, and it may have been for this reason she did not react to the active mycoplasma infection that was mentioned.

Cody had tons of ear and sinus infections, very serious ones. He had pneumonia a lot as well, but streptococcal pneumonia has the word strep in it, so that has to be the culprit of PANDAS.

Dr. T put Cody on antibiotics for his sinuses.

What Liz did not realize at the time was that she had just learned of a vital piece of the puzzle—a corner piece, perhaps. But not realizing its significance, she set it aside.

RESULTS FROM MICHELLE AND ADAM'S PSYCH EVALUATIONS

The results from the psychological testing ordered by Dr. Brunner were in, and Liz went to Mission Clinic to discuss the results. The therapist let Liz know that Adam and Michelle had both had been diagnosed with attachment disorders.

Though these issues were common among children who had been in the state's custody, the diagnoses did not make sense to Liz. In the five years since their adoption, they had both acclimated very well to their new family.

---

14 Streptococcal pneumonia usually causes ear infections and sinus infections.
15 Scientists call walking pneumonia caused by mycoplasma "atypical" because of the unique features of the bacteria itself. Some factors that make it atypical include milder symptoms and natural resistance to medicines that would normally treat bacterial infections.

"Why did they not have these disorders when they first came to live with us?" Liz wanted to know. "They went to therapy right away, and I was told that they were fine. How is it that they developed attachment disorders five years later?"

"Sometimes that happens during adolescence," the therapist explained.

Liz felt nauseous. She took a deep breath and asked, "What can I do?"

In answer to that question, a four-hundred-page book on attachment disorders arrived in the mail.

To make up for her possible shortcomings as a mother, Liz worked through numerous uncomfortable and time-consuming attachment exercises. These exercises only succeeded in making Michelle anxious and Adam confused, but Liz was determined not to let her kids down by skipping the exercises.

RESULTS FROM CODY'S PSYCH EVALUATION

Meanwhile, Cody's therapist at Mission Clinic agreed that Cody had experienced significant trauma during solitary confinement. But he neither understood nor agreed with the PANS/PANDAS diagnosis.

When Liz entered his office, he was reading up on PANDAS on Wikipedia and launched with a disheartening, "So... this PANDAS is a controversial diagnosis..."

Do medical professionals refer to Wikipedia for information?

That aside, it frustrated Liz that there was so little agreement among medical professionals regarding this condition.

Unless Cody's myriad of psychiatric symptoms were caused by a variety of different infections, how could they come and go as they do? Likewise, if strep could lead to OCD, anxiety, and a host of other symptoms, maybe other infections caused different psychiatric symptoms. Different strains of the flu cause different physical symptoms, so it made sense to Liz that it would be the same in children with PANS.

Why was it so difficult to grasp this concept? Was it controversial because it could prove that infections were the root of most—if not all—psychiatric diagnoses?

Was the $300 billion in annual revenues from the psych industry preventing this connection from being made?

There is no way I'm the first to piece this together. I'm not a doctor, but I certainly recognize a business deal and profit margins when I see them.

There's got to be a dollar sign somewhere on the puzzle box!

A TUMULTUOUS START TO THE NINTH GRADE

Cody had been in therapy all summer for trauma. The detention center trauma and death of a baby were a lot to deal with, but he seemed to be making some progress.

When he began having throat tics shortly after starting back to school, though, Liz grew alarmed. The year before, Cody's unusual blinking turned out to be a sign of a flare coming on. Plus, he had finished his prescription for the antibiotics Dr. T. had given him.

Liz also realized that Cody had been labeled a "bad kid," so she thought it could just be nervousness about being back to school.

But it was not just nerves. It did not take long for things to go from bad to unbearable.

Within a few weeks, Cody had become a completely different person again. Hoping Vanderbilt hospital could help this time, Liz took him to the emergency room. After learning that Cody had lost fourteen pounds within the past few months, the ER doctor quickly assessed his white-coated tongue and red throat and referred Cody to the Infectious Disease Department.

Liz knew they would not do anything other than send Cody to psych. She asked for more antibiotics that would target his sinuses, but they refused.

They say the definition of insanity is doing the same things and expecting a different result. I'm done with Vanderbilt!

On their way home from the hospital, Cody had a complete mental breakdown. It was like something possessed him.

Going in and out of the episode, Cody cried, saying, "Mom, you said this wouldn't happen again!"

Liz could barely see the road for her tears. As Cody started talking about people with guns who were following them, Liz knew her son had lost touch with reality completely.

TURNING TO DR. TRIFILETTI FOR ANSWERS

If anybody would have the answers, she felt certain it would be Dr. T. To Liz's relief, he understood the urgency of the situation and agreed to see them immediately. They packed the car and drove the seventeen hours to New Jersey.

This time, Kelsey went along to help. It took them both to keep Cody from jumping out of the car or running away altogether as he was in full "fight or flight" mode.

"There is nobody else who can help me comprehend what is happening to my son. Can you explain the results of Cody's Cunningham Panel to me?" Liz asked as soon as they sat down in Dr. T's office. She handed him the labs.[16]

---

16 **A note from the author:** If you don't already do this, you may want to ask your doctor for permission to record your consultation. The laws may vary from state to state regarding making audio recordings at your doctor's office. Recording the consultations allows you to listen again and catch details you may have missed during the visit. The voice note function on a smartphone works well for this purpose. Dr. T agreed for me to record our sessions.

"Hmm… It's like Cody has PANDAS *plus*. But what's the plus?" Dr. T leaned back in his chair. "He seems still in the early phases, though, so it should be reversible… possibly without IVIG."

Liz squeezed Cody's hand. Then her stomach dropped.

If this is what the early phase is like, how will we ever make it through the more advanced stages?

She set her notepad on the table.

"This is the second time Cody has essentially turned into someone else altogether, right before my eyes," she told Dr. T. "When he's like this, I'm not really talking to Cody. It's as if he's not there."

"Indeed," Dr. T told Liz, "PANS/PANDAS sufferers can dissociate when they have infections—meaning they don't know what they are doing. It's like an out-of-body experience."

Dr. T turned his chair to face her, letting the gravity of the next statement sink in. "But even when they are not themselves, they are still held responsible for what they do."

"Okay, let me get this straight: Because my child has a rare autoimmune disease, he can contract an infection and end up in a dissociative state? And then, while he is in this state, he can do something he's unaware of that may land him in prison for the rest of his life?"

Although this confirmed what she had personally witnessed in Cody, Liz was furious. She continued, "And all this would happen because no doctor or therapist where we live knows what the hell to do?"

The reality was sinking in. Her child's entire future depended on her understanding his condition.

She needed to work with Dr. T as closely as possible to solve Cody's case. Trying to think of what the *plus* could be, Liz asked,

"Would the trauma of being locked up in a cell for weeks have made things much worse?"

"Of course."

The third corner of the puzzle had just been dug out from the pile.

"What do I do about school until we get this figured out? They're all over me for truancy."

"Cody should *not* be in school until we get to the bottom of this," Dr. T assured her.

Liz asked Dr. T to write a note for school, which he agreed to do. She picked up her notebook again. "Why doesn't Cody get fevers?"

"In PANDAS, it is believed that the part of the immune system that is meant to trigger the fever center becomes misdirected and 'tickles' the amygdala—the rage center of the body," he explained.

The amygdala. That is connected to criminal behavior.

"So, instead of getting fevers, they have rage?"

"Exactly. And during those flares, they can have incredible strength."

Throwing movie theater chairs, smashing a laptop in half, the broken clavicle during the wrestling match...

"He seems so scared, and I don't understand why. Look at his pupils—they are *huge*. What can we do?"

"Run extensive genetic labs," Dr. T added confidently. "This sounds like a medical issue. I mean, what other explanation is there for someone to change *that* dramatically within a matter of hours and then get better? It has to be an infection."

Indeed, there was no other explanation.

That day, Dr. T ordered extensive genetic testing, started Cody on an antiviral again, and added a new, longer course of antibiotics targeting his sinuses.

After merely two weeks on the antibiotics and antivirals Dr. T had prescribed, Cody's symptoms had improved, though much differently than the way they had with IVIG the year before. His eyes were brighter, he seemed more connected and his face looked healthier.

Liz posted on the PANDAS Facebook page: "I am watching a miracle happen. My son's symptoms are literally unwinding in front of my eyes. I wonder if I have ever even met the real Cody."

Medical treatment works. I've seen again with my own eyes.

GETTING A NEW DOG

It was close to Cody's birthday, so Liz took Cody to the Humane Society. "Happy birthday, son! Let's go pick out a dog for you."

Cody *loved* animals, but he did not share Liz's excitement about getting a new dog. He reminded Liz that his pets always die. "Rusty, my guinea pigs, my bearded dragons—everything dies. And you know I took really good care of them."

She had to admit that Cody was right. Despite having taken excellent care of his pets over the years, they all died an early death. "Come on," Liz said. "Let's give it another shot."

The fear of losing another pet seemed to disappear the moment Cody spotted a black lab. Cody was in love. Buzz and Cody were soon inseparable.

But not long after, Buzz started coughing and drooling. Concerned that Buzz might be sick, and Cody could catch what he has—or worse yet, that Buzz could die—Liz rushed him to the veterinarian. "Please, we need to keep him healthy," Liz insisted.

Buzz tested negative for everything the veterinarian could think of, but he prescribed him ten days of antibiotics.

To everyone's relief, Buzz seemed to get better.

REMOVING ALL DISTRACTIONS

Liz was determined to remove all distractions, so she called a meeting with Mark. Two of Mark's older children had moved in, plus there seemed to be an endless stream of visitors coming through the home to see baby Hunter. It had to stop.

Liz also figured that it would be good for Mark to work less and focus more on his health. He had developed irritable bowel syndrome, had exorbitantly high cholesterol, and his hepatitis C had returned.

"I appreciate all you have done for us, but it's time for you to find another place for your family to live," she told Mark. "You can come in a few days a week to help out if that would work for you."

Mark understood. Soon after the talk, he and his family moved out.

Liz could not risk Cody being exposed to infections now that he seemed to be getting better. She was beginning to understand that not all infections responded to the same antibiotics. She could not risk any more unnecessary exposure, though.

But it was not only Cody who needed her attention. Michelle was rapidly becoming more defiant, and Adam seemed to have moved to another planet altogether. Her kids.

Liz needed to clear out anything and everyone that could distract her from figuring out exactly what was going on, why she, her children, and everyone around them seemed to be sick.

All she knew for sure was that something was terribly wrong in their home.

CHAPTER 11

Misdirected Immune Response

LOOKING FOR WAYS TO HELP CODY AT SCHOOL

Liz had turned in the note from Dr. Trifiletti stating that Cody was excused from school. Still, the principal left Liz a voicemail asking for a doctor's note. He scheduled a meeting to address the issue.

"I've provided the note from the neurologist who founded the PANDAS Institute," Liz said confidently before they had even taken their seats. "And I've been working with the central office to get Cody approved for homebound schooling."

"As for your request: It seems as if they've officially denied it," the school psychologist spoke on behalf of the group. "And we'll need a note from a *local* doctor."

"What?!" Liz was taken off guard. She had managed to comply with all of their rules, completed all of their forms, and supplied the necessary documentation. "Why was it denied?"

"The notes say that PANDAS is a form of OCD, and it doesn't meet the requirements for homebound schooling," she explained.

What notes? Probably Wikipedia.

Realizing that no one in the room had the authority to change the decision, Liz asked for an IEP.[17]

"Perhaps Cody could get a reduced workload," she suggested.

The psychologist agreed to set up the testing. After the testing was completed, the group reconvened.

"Cody doesn't have any learning disabilities," the psychologist reported. "Quite the opposite. He's a very smart young man."

Since the psychologist had worked with Cody for several days in a row and several hours at a time, Liz enquired whether she saw any signs of ODD.

"Not at all. He was very respectful and tried very hard."

"Did he show any signs of ADHD?"

"I didn't notice any. He got up a few times to walk around because of anxiety, but not that often. Once he sat down to work, he stayed focused until he was finished."

"I'm so grateful you could see who Cody really is," Liz said. "Did you notice any other disorders?"

"Other than the anxiety I mentioned? None that I could see."

Liz was relieved at the news. The last time Cody saw his therapist at Mission Clinic, the therapist said Cody had dissociation, OCD, and supposed conversion disorder.

So, it's not just me saying that medical treatment is working.

"Do you think he has any brain damage?" Liz asked.

"Well, I'm not a medical doctor so I can't say for sure, but his cognitive function appears to be just fine."

---

17   An individualized education program (IEP) is a document developed for a US public school child who is eligible for special education, which can mandate a reduced workload, varied schedule, and support with academics (if needed).

Even though Cody did not qualify for an IEP, it had been worth the testing to learn that Cody may not have permanent brain damage from the chronic inflammation.

Liz thanked the group for their time before closing her binder, and she headed home. For now, Cody would have just as much work to complete as anyone in the school who was not dealing with PANS/PANDAS.

BACK TO MISSION CLINIC FOR A DOCTOR'S NOTE

To avoid being charged with truancy for not sending Cody to school, Liz reached out to Dr. Brunner, Cody's pediatrician at Mission Clinic. He was not available, but Liz was told they could see the physician's assistant.

After reading what Dr. T had written, the PA agreed to write a note for school. It was only for a few days, but it helped.

Liz preferred not to send Cody to school until his flares were under control. The risk was too high. Homeschool did not feel like an option either.

What Liz needed was more time, and she needed to continue her search for a local doctor who was willing to work in partnership with Dr. T. For now, it would help if she could understand the lab results from Dr. T, so Liz asked the PA if he could help her interpret those. She pulled out the most recent set of labs from Dr. T and her spreadsheet for comparison.

Maybe if the PA sees these results, he might agree to be the local connection we need for continuing Cody's treatment.

"Cody got better with the IVIG and then again with antivirals," she explained. "And now, he's doing even better with antibiotics for sinuses."

She pointed to the results of Cody's pneumococcal titer test. "Would those numbers for the *Streptococcus pneumoniae* go down with antibiotics if he didn't have an active infection?"

"No, they wouldn't," he affirmed Liz's hunch. "You need to go to infectious disease... and immunology. You guys need a team."

A team is exactly what Cody needs! A team could help us solve this thousand-piece puzzle. I'm not stopping till this puzzle is put together!

"I'll set up the referrals and personally follow up to make sure you get in ASAP," the PA promised.

Dr. Brunner was not nearly as enthusiastic about the PA's referrals. He squashed the plan and only referred Cody to an endocrinologist for his high thyroid antibodies.

Liz vented to Cody's therapist during their next session at Mission Clinic. He seemed to care about Cody and was trying to help him process the trauma from the juvenile detention center. But the therapist did not seem to think that Dr. Brunner's approach was an issue.

Maybe he thinks I have Munchausen's!

Unbeknownst to Liz, the therapist had forwarded Cody's lab results to another physician at Mission Clinic for a second opinion.

During their follow-up appointment, the therapist told Liz that the other doctor had explained to him that it was Cody's IgG that was high, not his IgM.[18] What's more, she learned that he thought the pneumococcal titer test did not mean what she had been told that it meant. The therapist was told that Cody did not

---

18 Both immunoglobulin G (IgG) and immunoglobulin M (IgM) are antibodies produced by the immune system to fight against infections. Simplistically stated, high IgM numbers indicate a current infection, while immunoglobin G only shows up well into or *after* the infection, when the new antibodies (IgM) are no longer present.

have any current medical problems and that he should not be on antibiotics.

No wonder Dr. Brunner wouldn't help us! And who is this mystery doctor that the therapist contacted? It sounds like the physicians all read from the same script!

ASSEMBLING A TEAM

The PA's suggestion to have a team work on Cody's case was brilliant, and if it meant Liz would convene a team on her own, she would do that. As for the referrals they needed to gain access to specialists, Liz was delighted to learn that, with a small copayment, she could schedule appointments with specialists. She would not need a referral after all.

Liz began making a wish list of physicians. She was determined to get Cody in to see all the specialists she had heard the doctors mention over the years of trying to find a solution to PANDAS: immunology, ENT, infectious disease, lung (because of the *Mycoplasma pneumoniae* infection, which she still needed to research further), genetics, and endocrinology. And they needed a new pediatrician. She was resolved to go see anyone she thought may be able to help.

She would ask each of them questions only related to their specialties and then attempt to put the pieces together herself.

Within two days, Liz had several different specialist visits scheduled, plus one with Dr. T to review Cody's genetic test results, which had just arrived.

DRAFTING A MEDICAL BRIEF

In light of all that had transpired around the mishandling of Cody's medical care, Liz had decided to hold Dr. Meneely accountable. She would be filing a medical malpractice suit against him, and she needed a medical expert to provide testimony in court.

Tennessee medical malpractice laws required that the expert testimony against Dr. Meneely comes from a doctor within the state or states immediately neighboring it.

As Liz flipped through Cody's huge stack of records dating back to the day he was born, she came up with an idea that would kill two birds with one stone.

As I draft the synopsis of Cody's medical history for the malpractice case, I can also create a master timeline for these specialists. Psych symptoms and behaviors will be in a separate column. I have got to learn words other than PANS/PANDAS and strep.

Once Liz started, she could not stop. And by day three, she began to notice a pattern emerging.

Cody got an infection as a baby and it never left.

She continued reading, typing, and referencing. The pieces seemed to connect perfectly to form some of the edges around the puzzle.

By day five, Liz had mapped out Cody's entire medical history in a twenty-three-page document organized for each of the specialists.[19]

Medical diagnoses such as possible viral syndrome, possible influenza, pharyngitis with no strep, high fevers, sinusitis, and bilateral pneumonia mixed in with some hearing problems at school, night terrors, and decreased appetite had evolved over the years into psychiatric terms: ADHD, possible ADD, possible ODD, anxiety disorder, and OCD.

---

19   **A note from the author:** While I was able to map out most of Cody's symptoms from birth, early handwritten records were difficult to decipher, and I would later discover important details that I had missed upon first reading.

Over time, Cody's fevers got lower and the medications changed from antibiotics like Zithromax, Rocephin, Cefzil, and amoxicillin to psychiatric drugs like Concerta, Vyvanse, Adderall, and Zoloft.

Liz thought back to Dr. T's explanation that Cody's rage center, instead of his fever center, was activated during infections.

Was this how Cody's immune response became misdirected?

Liz knew full well that the immune system did not have a personality or logic of its own. The brain responded to stimuli and initiated or maintained biological systems. But to unravel the complexities involved, she put that aside and in a somewhat radical—desperate?—approach, she imagined herself as the immune system.

If she were the immune system and had to solve this problem, what would she do?

If I had been activating high fevers and many other physical symptoms for years but found no relief, I would change my strategy as well. Cody's immune system isn't wrong—it's absolutely right! It's not broken—it's brilliant! My son's immune response had slowly changed its tactic. And why wouldn't it? If what it was doing wasn't working, of course it would try something different.

Maybe she was going too far, but she considered how ingenious it was that the immune system started setting off the part of the brain that caused behaviors—getting attention from parents and teachers that the fevers had not. It was doing everything in its power to fight the infection.

The ADHD, the jumping around in class—each behavior was ultimately screaming: "Help me, please!"

The OCD was Cody's brain's way of trying to put everything in perfect order outside of his body because something inside was completely out of order.

The separation anxiety developed because if anyone was going to figure out what was wrong, it would be Mom or Dad—and his subconsciousness was clinging to that fact.

The night terrors were a reaction to the monstrous infection attacking his brain.

The anxiety appeared from knowing that if the infection was not addressed soon, something horrible was going to happen.

The paranoia that someone would get him resulted from the fact that something already had him.

The solitude he had compulsively pursued by running away and finding quiet places in the woods was his innate way of protecting his loved ones from exposure.

The creation of panic rooms in case of an attack was because he was actively being attacked.

The ODD was brought on by his fury because even his mother was not able to help him.

Each of these patterns became sections of the jigsaw puzzle that were connecting to reveal snippets of the bigger picture.

Why hasn't anyone noticed this pattern before?

Most kids with PANDAS have high Streptococcus pneumoniae *titers, but Cody's are even higher than most. Are all of these symptoms related to that?*

These antibodies are the only common denominator.

Liz was more convinced than ever that if she did not figure out a way to kill the infection, it would kill Cody.

AVOIDING A CATASTROPHE

Dr. Meneely had broken Cody's immune system by not treating the infections properly when he still had fevers and other traditional signs of infection.

The more Liz realized that if the behaviors she had witnessed thus far were only a *tickling* of the amygdala, the more she understood the dire emergency of their situation.

What would happen if his amygdala was under total attack? Liz needed to stay focused; she had to stop this misdirected immune response before its aim hit Cody's amygdala dead center.

The medical malpractice suit became far less important as Liz shifted her focus to avoiding a catastrophe. If she were to sue anyone, it would probably be Judge Guffee.

LIZ IS FEELING SICK

On the way to the spa the next day, Liz felt a chill go up her spine—the first sign of her coming down with something. She immediately called John.

"I need to bring the kids to your house," she said, explaining that she might be getting sick. "I don't want to expose them to anything—especially Cody."

After ten days, the chills finally tapered off, but then her neck started tightening.

If I go to the hospital, they likely won't recognize these symptoms anyway. And if I caught something from Cody? Well, he's still alive. I can ride it out.

Liz figured she could have caught pneumonia from Cody, though she did not have any of the normal symptoms of pneumonia—no coughing. No fever.

Is my fever center broken too?

She could not remember having a fever since the time her family had become deathly ill when Steven moved in with them, about twelve years ago.

The following morning, Liz could barely open her jaw.

Chills, a tight neck, and now lockjaw? What is going on?

With one mysterious horror after another, Liz felt that she was in a bad movie that had no end.

CHAPTER 12

A Team of One

SEEING AN INFECTIOUS DISEASE DOCTOR

An infectious disease doctor at Vanderbilt was one of the first appointments. The doctor walked in with a fellow.[20]

Liz strategically asked the doctor her questions but was not getting anywhere. The doctor seemed guarded. Still, he was keen to let Liz know that the labs showed Cody's response to the pneumococcal vaccine and that they did not indicate a current infection.[21]

The script again.

Liz wished that as an infectious disease doctor, he could help her connect some of the pieces of the puzzle. She knew these

---

20 A fellow is a medical professional who is in the process of being trained in a medical specialty.

21 **A note from the author:** I did not bother letting the doctor know that, somehow, Cody had never gotten the series of vaccines. I suspect it's because he had already had pneumonia several times before he was two, but I cannot be sure.

numbers held clues. The doctor walked out to order an HIV[22] test for Cody.

An HIV test?!

Liz showed her copy of the spreadsheet of Cody's labs to the fellow and asked, "Do you think it's odd that Cody started antibiotics for his sinuses and these numbers went down?"

He paused before asking how the doctor Cody had seen knew to run that test.

That look of intrigue again, now we are getting somewhere.

After Cody's test was over, Liz remembered the promise she had made to herself. She would ask one question unrelated to PANS/PANDAS that this specialist may be able to answer. "How do viruses work in combination with streptococcal pneumonia?"[23] she asked him.

He perked up. "Everyone carries *Streptococcus pneumoniae* bacterium in their nose," he explained. "It is part of the normal microorganisms that live in your body, but if a *pathogenic*—a disease-causing—strain of the bacterium is present, and if a virus is inhaled, then the environment is ideal for flu or flu-like symptoms."

More pieces of the puzzle were clicking in place but others seemed to be dropping off the table.

That's what happens all over Cody's body! But there are twenty-three strains on that test Dr. Tran. How will I know which one could be causing his "psych flu"?

The doctor changed the topic, observing that he had never seen anyone on antivirals other than HIV-positive patients.

---

22 Human immunodeficiency viruses (HIV) are known to cause acquired immunodeficiency syndrome (AIDS). One of the known treatments for HIV is antiviral medications.

23 Streptococcal pneumonia refers to the infection, whereas *Streptococcus pneumoniae* is the Latin term that refers to the bacterium that causes the infection.

"Please do not take Cody's antivirals away," she pleaded. "They are helping. Please!" The doctor stood in silence looking baffled.

Maybe I sounded too desperate, I hope he doesn't think I'm crazy.

Liz's mind was spinning. She thought about the Justina Pelletier case in which a hospitalist had decided that Justina did not have the rare genetic disorder her doctor and parents believed she had.

They had contacted child protective services to mandate the treatment they had chosen for her. After more than 16 months in state custody—much of it in a locked psychiatric ward, the traumatized teen was returned to her family. She was still in a wheelchair, and still sick from her disease.

I don't want our family to become victims of medical kidnapping.

"Well, if you have a doctor who will continue to prescribe and monitor him on them," the doctor replied, "I guess they won't hurt."

LINING UP THE PIECES

After a marathon of doctor's visits and with several more to attend, Liz was emotionally spent. But Cody's symptoms were escalating again. Once it started, it was hard to stop.

This happened each time he completed a prescription of antibiotics.[24] Liz had to think fast to figure out what to do to help with de-escalating the symptoms.

That night, Liz tossed and turned trying to come up with the answer to what was causing Cody's PANS/PANDAS.

Why aren't the antibiotics killing whatever this is?

---

24 **A note from the author:** Over time, I came to learn that this "honeymoon period" of reduced or no symptoms during a round of antibiotics differed. It varied between two days and two weeks. Let me not get ahead of myself, though. I'll tell you more about this process in chapter 20. The point is, I was only seeing the honeymoon period of antibiotics because Cody kept stopping then restarting as I could get more.

She had learned a lot of new words from all of the doctors and felt braver than ever before, but she needed to maintain her confidence because no one seemed to have the answer she desperately needed. She slipped into her pj's.

I might as well get comfortable. This might be another long night. I can do this!

From the box filled with Cody's medical records, Liz pulled out the ones from the fall of 2010, when Cody had his sudden onset of OCD—when the term PANDAS entered their world.

She combed through the records, line by line, looking for insights.

That night, she noticed something she had not been aware of before: Strep was not the only diagnosis Cody was found to have during that fateful visit to the Vanderbilt emergency room. He also had pneumonia.

What? They didn't tell me he had pneumonia too!

Liz grabbed the stack of records from Dr. Meneely's office, turning to the visit two weeks prior to that event. Sure enough, the records showed that Cody had group A strep *and* pneumonia.

Dr. Meneely did not tell us that Cody had pneumonia. The fact that Cody not only had strep but also pneumonia at the time of the acute onset of PANDAS must mean something. Maybe I should take him back to the lung doctor so she can take another look.

Liz finally drifted off to sleep right before the sun came up.

CHAPTER 13

Superbug

AN IMPORTANT PIECE OF THE PUZZLE

Liz awoke to her alarm and a million unanswered questions. After breakfast, she dove into her research.

Okay, you can wrap your mind around this; don't give up.

She flipped open her laptop, inhaled deeply, and became one with the lab results. She soon learned that *Streptococcus pneumoniae* was first isolated by Louis Pasteur in the saliva from a child who had died of rabies.

Rabies! She laughed. *That explains a lot!*

Streptococcus pneumoniae can be transmitted through sneezing, coughing, and direct contact. Plus, it is highly contagious.

Cody got his first ear infection at three months old, but he hadn't gone to daycare by then. How did he get it in the first place?

After much searching, Liz stumbled upon an article by Dr. Michael Pichichero that caught her attention. It was titled "Ear infection superbug discovered to be resistant to all pediatric antibiotics."

Liz remembered a nurse friend of hers explaining that a superbug is a kind of bug with the superpower of suppressing its victim's immune system so the victim can neither fight the bug—nor anything else.

Liz could not shake the feeling that a superbug may be playing the role of a villain in this movie that her family was living.

In the same article, Dr. Pichichero warned that, while it may never happen, the medical profession must consider that 19A—the multi-drug resistant strain of *Streptococcus pneumoniae*—has been known to show up as a bacterial ear infection, but it could spread to other parts of the body. It could invade the lungs and bloodstream where it could lead to pneumonia or meningitis that were only treatable with antibiotics not approved for use in children.

Cody's 19A is through the roof! Maybe this is it? Maybe this is the culprit!

She recalled details from Cody's medical timeline.

From ear infection to eye infection to pneumonia—it's been almost fourteen years now. Surely, it's spread everywhere it possibly can in Cody.

The article went on to explain that the only antibiotic that killed the 19A strain was Levaquin, and while it had been approved for adults, there was a warning on its label against use in children. The researcher had tried it anyway, and it worked.

If 19A was the root of Cody's problems, then it should respond to Levaquin.

Cody had been given all the typical pediatric antibiotics before the age of two, and the records proved that none of them had worked.

This has to mean that Cody has a resistant strain like 19A. This could be the answer!

All Liz had to do was get Cody a prescription for a drug not intended for children from a doctor who did not believe anything was medically wrong with him in the first place.

Well, now I can sleep peacefully.

Realizing that Cody might have a superbug, Liz was relieved that she had not been sending Cody to school, or else he could be spreading this bug. Liz emailed Dr. T for another appointment before closing her laptop for the night.

I need to see if Cody's 19A has changed again. I don't care if I do go to jail for truancy, but I will not be guilty of starting an epidemic.

SEARCHING FOR MORE ANSWERS

Liz had many questions that kept her going in her search for answers. Questions such as how the professors in medical school could educate medical students about the symptoms of bacterial strains that had not even been discovered. They cannot. It is impossible.

As new studies become available, they get published in medical journals. And for articles to get published in such journals, they go through a strenuous review process to ensure the research is solid.

Liz discovered that she could access these articles on PubMed— an online library of peer-reviewed medical articles.

Textbooks are outdated. Simply asking Google for answers? Not reliable.

To guide her in her search, Liz not only relied on insights from everything she had read and studied over the last several months, but she would also build upon what she learned in college and post-college education.

Liz would also rely on the confidence she had gained from being a spa owner who created her own skincare line and drafted a new theory on the development of cellulite. For her current research, PubMed would have to serve as her constantly updated textbook.

She also relied on prayer, asking God for continued guidance in her search to find out what was wrong with her son.

It did not take long for Liz to realize that Cody's situation was worse than she had thought before. She wrestled with the dilemma of what could happen if a doctor prescribed Levaquin and it did not kill all the 19A.

Would the 19A become resistant to Levaquin? Could all these antibiotics make any other bugs Cody might have resistant? Could they become superbugs too?

Getting a "super superbug" named after her son was not her definition of success.

CHAPTER 14
Genetic Testing

MICHELLE'S NEW SYMPTOM

Liz needed to know if 19A—the multi-drug resistant strain of *Streptococcus pneumoniae*—had spread from Cody's ears and sinuses to his lungs. Where else could it go?

She tried to schedule an appt with Dr. Pichichero, the researcher who discovered the resistance of this strain. If anyone would know, it would be him. While Liz searched and searched to find a number, Michelle came in. She was visibly nervous.

"Mom, there is something weird by my ear. It really hurts. Can you see what it is?" Michelle leaned down to show Liz a big, red cyst-like boil that festered behind her earlobe. It was warm to the touch.

The last two years of Michelle's life flashed in front of Liz: isolation, ADHD, sleep disorder, anxiety, high heart rate, and headaches. Most recently, there was the ODD, behavior that was completely uncharacteristic of her sweet and sensitive daughter.

Could Michelle have contracted 19A from Cody? Dr. T. kept referring to Cody's struggles as neuropsychiatric symptoms, symptoms of the brain. Could Michelle have them too?

Liz went to get a warm compress for Michelle's ear. As the water ran, she got lost in thought.

Michelle's fever center isn't broken. And if she had caught 19A from Cody, it couldn't have been until she was seven years old, when she and Adam were adopted. Plus, Michelle didn't have PANDAS. Or did she?

Liz thought back to the terrible staph infection Michelle had gotten at a camp a few weeks after moving in.

Had she picked it up at camp, or had she caught that from Cody as well? Michelle and Cody had different genetics. They each also had unique physical and neuropsychiatric symptoms. But how was it possible that they also shared some of the same symptoms? Did 19A cause ODD, or was ODD just one of the symptoms of 19A?

If this were the case, Michelle and Cody should not be disciplined for ODD any more than they should be for developing a boil.

Liz began to internalize these concepts.

No mother would demand that her child "reduce his fever immediately," nor would a father tell his child to "quit coughing." A child is not punished for disobedience when they are unable to immediately heal from the flu.

We have always turned to doctors to help reduce a fever or ease a cough. But the rules have changed. The symptoms have changed. The infections have changed. Now, we need to be able to turn to doctors to reduce defiance and calm obsessions.

More pieces of this puzzle seemed to be connecting.

TREATING PSYCHOLOGICAL SYMPTOMS MEDICALLY

So far, Liz had always believed that Michelle's childhood trauma and hormonal changes were responsible for her symptoms of ODD. But after learning of 19A and seeing the boil—a physical sign of an infection—she took Michelle to see Dr. Brunner.

She was hoping he would give her antibiotics for the boil, which, if she were right, could help alleviate her ODD. Liz was convinced that if she could get rid of the organism causing the boil, then all the related neuropsychiatric symptoms would resolve themselves as well.

Dr. Brunner readily prescribed antibiotics for the boil, but Liz had unsuccessfully tried to convince him to send in a sample for analysis.

LABILE EMOTIONS AND TOURETTE'S SYNDROME

When Dr. Trifiletti emailed the results of Cody's most recent labs, Liz saw that Cody's *Streptococcus pneumoniae* titers were increasing again.

Maybe he has that genetic disorder Dr. T had mentioned that made it hard for him to fight infections.

Dr. T included a note that the genetic testing would be in soon. Liz was particularly interested to see if Cody may have some type of genetic disorder that may be playing a role.

In the few weeks it had taken to get the labs, things had started to unravel. That evening, Cody was already having what Liz has learned to be labile emotions—emotions that do not match the situation—his Tourette's, a new symptom, was particularly unnerving, and he was agitated and anxious. Emotionally, Cody was all over the map.

It was a Friday night. Liz could not wait for the next appointment with Dr. T. Something had to be done at once. But she was worn out trying to learn all she had to keep her kids well.

God, this is too much for one person. Too much.

ON A MISSION TO GET LEVAQUIN

Late that night, Cody cut a deep wound in his finger. In a normal situation, a parent would have rushed their child straight to the emergency room for stitches, but Liz considered her next moves carefully.

Cody's paranoia had kicked in, and if they saw him in this state, they would put him in the psychiatric hospital again. And he was the worst at night. I can take him tomorrow.

She cleaned his wound and taped it together with butterfly stitches so that she could buy herself more time to think.

The next morning Cody came downstairs with his hand over his left eye.

"Mom, my eye is burning like fire."

Considering that the infection might be escalating, Liz carefully taped a piece of gauze over his left eye.

Cody's vision improves when he is on antibiotics. Now his eye is burning after a few weeks of stopping. Is the resistant colony behind his left eye?

Dr. Pichichero's article stated that the only antibiotic that killed 19A was Levaquin. Instinctively, Liz needed to get some for Cody.

MAYBE THIS IS THE ANSWER

With Cody in this state, Liz decided to try a different hospital. She took him to Williamson Medical Center.

"You have a really interesting story here," the PA said as he walked into the exam room. He held up Cody's intake form. "I see that you guys have worked with specialists from all over the country. What brings you in today?"

Liz gave him an abbreviated spreadsheet that documented the ups and downs of Cody's *Streptococcus pneumoniae* titers. Next, she showed him the article about superbugs and pointed out the fact that Cody's labs indicate the presence of 19A in his system.

"This researcher has found that the only antibiotic that works to fight 19A, the multi-drug resistant strain of *Streptococcus pneumoniae* is Levaquin," Liz said, pointing it out in the article.

He turned to look at Liz, "Do you know you're asking me to give your son something that could rupture his tendons?" the PA asked bluntly.

When Cody was at his worst, Liz could not do anything to stop the intense anxiety and compulsions that ultimately involved police intervention. Given the choice between solitary confinement in the children's county prison for weeks or a ruptured tendon, she would take the latter—though she hoped it would not come to that.

The PA examined Cody and found that, in addition to the psych symptoms, Cody complained of tenderness on his nose, and his eyebrow and temple were red and hot.

If only we could see if 19A is behind his eyes...

They left with a prescription for Levaquin and discharge papers that listed "acute sinusitis" as the diagnosis.

At the pharmacy, when the pharmacist discussed the possible side effects of the new medicine, he said nothing about ruptured tendons. Liz asked him about it, and he assured her that it will not happen.

"Cody's the size of a grown man," he smiled, "not a small boy!"

It struck Liz how mature her son might appear to others. Even though he was only fourteen, he was nearly six feet tall. But to Liz, Cody was still her little boy.

She gave him his first dose of Levaquin the minute they got home.

FEEDING THE RAGE

Cody's anger resurfaced the very next day.

It could take twenty-four hours for antibiotics to start working... right?

Liz was desperate for the Levaquin to work.

The fury did not subside. Instead, it escalated into an uncontrollable fit of rage in which Cody broke his toe.

Liz wondered if something was seriously wrong.

The antibiotics are supposedly killing the bacteria. But something seems to be feeding the rage!

Liz had read that when pneumonia bacteria died, they released ammonia.

Could it be that the ammonia was irritating Cody, turning him into the Hulk?

To neutralize the ammonia, Liz drew her son a warm Epsom salt bath. Amazingly, the bath seemed to wash away both the ammonia and his temper. Once out of the tub, Cody was relaxed and able to fall asleep.

He was so at peace that he slept for twenty-four hours. Liz checked on him often before finally waking him the following morning.

FEELING GOOD

Cody strolled into the living room and plopped down on the sofa. He looked around the sunlit room and smiled.

"Mom, I have never felt this good in my entire life."

Liz stared in disbelief. Not once has she seen Cody this relaxed on the sofa, calmly watching television without fidgeting and without having to constantly get up. Nor had he ever volunteered feeling so much better in a short amount of time. He just sat and enjoyed the shows. Liz feared that if she so much as moved a pinkie, she may awaken from this beautiful dream.

She and Cody watched television all day long, enjoying the time together. Liz was elated.

It is working! The Levaquin is killing the 19A!

GETTING THE GENETIC TEST RESULTS

By the following day, Cody's OCD and anxiety were almost gone. He was sweet, helpful, and friendly to his siblings, which gave Liz time to catch up on some emails.

Her inbox held the long-awaited results from Cody's extensive genetic testing. Dr. T reviewed the results as Liz sat in disbelief. She learned that Cody did not have the genetic predisposition for any of the symptoms he had displayed nor those of the diagnoses he had been given.

Based on Cody's genes, his medical situation should look entirely different.

If the issues are not rooted in Cody's genetic makeup, and since Michelle has different genes altogether, the cause has to be external. But what is it?

Do not let up. Think outside the box.

It seemed like resistant organisms were spreading like wildfires with no system in place to contain them.

Liz knew that to be true. She had a front-row seat to the chaos spreading all around her.

A SWIFT RETURN

Cody's symptoms returned swiftly and fiercely within a day of him taking his last dose of Levaquin. He was back in the garage cleaning, organizing, and arranging things in his lab until the wee hours of the morning.

Although Liz was disappointed by the regression, she did not feel nearly the same level of desperation that she had before.

Her theories had turned into a short-lived reality. She had seen Cody as symptom-free as he had ever been. Since she knew this feat was possible, she resolved to repeat it and make it stick.

Early the next morning when Liz walked into the kitchen, Cody was already up.

"Good morning, Mom. Look what I did for you." He opened the refrigerator door. The fridge was immaculate. Anything that was out of date had been discarded, the glass shelves were sparkling, and the jars were organized in the door by height. All the plastics were on the bottom shelf with the lids in perfect alignment. Any plastic that did not fit into the scheme had been placed in the kitchen sink.

Not only had Cody cleaned the refrigerator, but he had also cleaned the entire kitchen! "Wow, that looks wonderful…" Liz tried to hide her concern. It was great when kids did nice things for their parents, but when Cody did them, it meant something else altogether.

Where did all the food go?

Liz managed to find the ingredients to make everyone oatmeal. While they ate breakfast, Liz got as creative as possible with what she could find to pack their lunches for summer band camp.

"Could you make me a PB&J, please?" Michelle gave her an exaggerated smile of appreciation.

"Sure, honey." Liz grabbed the jar of peanut butter.

Wait a minute. It had been four days since Michelle had started her antibiotics, and she had not screamed or slammed a door once...

"How is that boil doing, honey? Is it going down?"

While the boil had not healed completely yet, it had gone down quite a bit and was not as red.

OFF TO SEE AN EAR, NOSE, AND THROAT DOCTOR

Wanting to find out if Cody had a bacterial colony in the cavity behind his eye, Liz made an appointment for Cody to see an ear, nose, and throat doctor. She carefully selected the abbreviated labs of Cody's MRI results and medical records to take with them.

She explained their story to the ENT about the IVIG, the antivirals, and the antibiotics that were making Cody better. "Dr. Trifiletti said that Cody's sinuses were 'raging,' and we needed to make sure they stayed clear. Maybe you might find a hidden bacterial colony."

"I see," he said. "Let's do a CAT scan to look at Cody's sinus cavities."

Please God, let us find this thing so that Cody can have the life you meant for him to have.

"I don't want to be responsible for creating some super superbug inside of Cody," she admitted. "Just in case five days of antibiotics killed most of it, but not all of it, would you please prescribe another round of Levaquin?"

They left with another two weeks' worth.

Within twenty-four hours, Cody was practically asymptomatic again. He could even ignore the coffee spoon that Liz left on the counter each morning to stir her second cup of coffee.

Two times is no coincidence—it's a confirmation.

But the antibiotics were numbered.

I have exactly two weeks—now thirteen days—to find this invisible, hidden pathogen that is wrecking our lives.

SEARCHING FOR A HIDDEN BACTERIAL COLONY

Liz stared at Cody's CAT scan for hours. She zeroed in on every structure behind Cody's eyes until she came across the ethmoid bone, which was a spongy bone where mucus was produced.

When the ENT called saying Cody's sinuses were clear, Liz was not disappointed. She knew she was getting closer.

Believe in yourself. You saw the relief with your own eyes. It is there, we just have not found it yet.

CHAPTER 15

A Broken Immune System

THE MOTIVATION OF A MOTHER

Now that Cody was on antibiotics, their lives resembled normal. The boys played well together that evening—it almost felt like a healthy household.

Liz took full advantage of the calm and took a relaxing shower. That was where the realization came to Liz: The various aspects of Cody's disease were not isolated. One led to another.

Each piece of this puzzle connected to another. And another. PANS/PANDAS seemed to encompass every specialty in the medical field. This was an overwhelming reality.

Liz did not know if she could ever do enough to help Cody. But she knew that she had something the doctors did not— *motivation*. The doctors she had seen locally may have had years of training and experience, but she was Cody's mother.

She was determined to find the answer.

SEEING AN IMMUNOLOGIST

Since PANDAS is an autoimmune disorder, Liz had included an immunologist in her list.[25] As part of her preparation for the meeting, she watched hours of videos on IVIG and the immune system.

She briefed the doctor on Cody's history, including his history with chronic ear infections and repeated episodes of both viral and bacterial pneumonia.

"What did his immunology workup show?" he asked.

Liz sighed. "Cody never had one." In thirteen years of taking Cody to Dr. Meneely for one infection after another, not once did he suggest that they do any immunology tests.

If I had moved Cody to a different pediatrician years ago, we probably wouldn't be sitting here trying to figure out which way the infection had gone and what damage had been done.

"Look, Cody has had *all* the strains of pneumonia. I realize that the strep pneumonia titer test wasn't intended for this purpose, but Cody did not get that series of vaccines, so they have to mean *something.*"

From her spreadsheets, Liz showed him how Cody's titer results have gone up and down over the past year, pointing out that they were on the rise again.

The immunologist looked pensive. "Did he improve with antibiotics?"

"Absolutely! Those ups and downs in the spreadsheet happen when he starts or stops antibiotics. I figure it's got to be connected. Cody got a little better when he was on antivirals, but he got *much* better with antibiotics, especially Levaquin." She continued, "He

---

25   An immunologist specializes in the immune system.

also got better with IVIG treatment, but that took a lot longer and wasn't as effective as having him on Levaquin."

"Well, IVIG works as an immunosuppressant, so some people with autoimmune diseases get better on it for that reason, but not because it is anti-infectious," he explained.

It took Liz a moment to process what the doctor just said: A therapy like IVIG can be helpful because it suppresses the immune system, but it does not kill the infection.

"What have they done to look for infection?" the immunologist wanted to know.

Liz explained that when Cody was at his worst, both MRIs had shown sinus issues.

"I wonder if there's some hidden bacterial colony that simply hasn't been found yet."

The doctor had blood drawn to conduct some tests, and they wrapped up the visit.

"Ms. Harris," he said as Liz headed out, "sometimes the only clue you get is when you accidentally stumble on a treatment that works. Then you work the problem backward."

AN ELEVATED WHITE BLOOD COUNT

Back at the spa, Liz was happy to see Gina, a long-time customer with a doctorate in psychology.

"Liz, it's good to see you," Gina smiled. "Hey, have you heard that the new *DSM* just came out? It took them over twelve years to agree on what new mental disorders to include—there are so many new ones that keep popping up! I think you'll find it interesting."

Liz had never looked into the *Diagnostic and Statistical Manual of Mental Disorders*, so after finishing Gina's treatment, she sat down at the computer to search. Liz did not get any further than hair pulling (trichotillomania), skin picking (excoriation), and cutting (non-suicidal self-injury disorder) before concluding that a veterinarian would have quickly recognized those behaviors as ones of infected animals.

To back her theory up, Liz found a study on OCD and depressive patients who showed elevated white blood counts—an immune response to an infection.

Why aren't patients with OCD at the doctor's office instead of at a psychologist?

Although she was only concerned with Cody's PANDAS, the other connections Liz was making during the process intrigued her.

CODY'S IMMUNOLOGY RESULTS

When Liz got the test results from Cody's immunology appointment, it showed that nothing was wrong with his immune system. This was on par with the immune function tests Dr. T had conducted.

Both Dr. T and the immunologist had confirmed that Cody's immunoglobulins were within normal levels.

Cody has neither genetic nor immunological abnormalities. Faulty immune system? Ruled out!

CHAPTER 16

Collecting Data

CAN THE BRAIN SENSE PAIN?

"Did your child have a lot of ear infections or pneumonia as a baby?" Liz polled the parents of children with PANDAS on their Facebook group one morning.

Within an hour, fifty members responded, all confirming her suspicion. Of course, it was not the scientific data the medical community needed, but it showed that a connection possibly existed.

Liz logged out of Facebook and began packing for their trip to Duke University in Durham, North Carolina. Cody had an appointment to see the Chief of Pediatric Infectious Diseases at Duke University Hospital.

Liz's mom, Carol, joined them for the trip.

With Cody faring well on Levaquin, they were able to spend quality time together. Liz listened as Carol and Cody took turns reading a book for his English class. Once Cody dozed off, Carol and Liz had a rare opportunity to catch up and talk about more than the children's health.

Carol shared with Liz some of the stress from her previous job working with patients with traumatic brain injuries and veterans with PTSD.[26]

"It was utterly exhausting," Carol admitted. "That's why I quit. The stress from that job made me physically sick. This might sound strange, but it felt like my brain was aching," she sighed.

"I know the brain doesn't have any pain receptors, so that doesn't make sense that my brain would hurt. But I could feel it."

"Well, Mom, you have to trust yourself. If it hurts, it hurts," Liz assured her. "It's strange that they didn't send you to see a neurologist. One of the things I've learned from this saga is that many psychiatric disorders are simply undiagnosed medical disorders. Imagine how much better folks would feel if only they got the right medical treatment…"

KELSEY IS HAVING SYMPTOMS

That evening, Kelsey sent Liz a picture of her thigh with a deep-red spot on it. "I thought you might want this for your research. Isn't it like the spot Cody got? It was just there when I woke up this morning!"

Liz tossed and turned that night. She lay in bed thinking of one thing after another from Kelsey's life, including pleurisy, ADHD, anxiety, chemical sensitivities—and many other symptoms that emerged over the past several years.

---

26 Post-traumatic stress disorder (PTSD) is a mental health condition that can develop after a person has experienced a traumatic event.

This is more than just an ear infection. Could this also be 19A? Or is there more to this? Whatever is causing these strange symptoms is all around me!

SEEING THE DOCTOR IN DURHAM

Liz awoke, surprised that she had slept. She was eager to meet this new infectious disease doctor. This woman had clinical experience with infections, unexplained fevers, meningitis, pneumonia, and viral diseases. Plus, she was doing research involving pediatric respiratory viral infections and vaccines.

Liz hoped it was worth traveling the eight hours to see her.

She soon found herself nervously explaining Cody's entire story yet again. "Cody's a great kid with a kind heart, but when he's sick, it is like something takes over. And until whatever it is has passed, he's simply is not himself. But even then, he's not quite his old self again."

"That sounds like a classic onset of PANDAS," the doctor stated resolutely.

For four years, Liz had known that Cody had PANDAS. She had seen the results of his Cunningham Panel. She had heard the diagnosis from several other doctors. Hearing those words from a world-renowned Chief of Pediatric Infectious Disease at an internationally recognized institution? It made it undeniable.

Liz also no longer felt afraid that she would lose her son because Vanderbilt did not agree with Dr. T, Dr. Karlton, or Dr. Latimer.

Of course, she would have given her right arm for Cody to have something other than this controversial and confusing disease.

The doctor turned her gaze to Cody. "We need you to let us know when you start to feel unwell—psychiatrically," the doctor said.

When Cody agreed, the doctors recommend that Liz works with psychiatrists to help manage symptoms.

"But then Cody wouldn't be able to tell me when he's not well. Psych meds would mask his symptoms," Liz explained, "Besides, when he's having a flare, there isn't a psych med out there strong enough to help him."

"And you feel able and willing to take care of him without psych meds?"

"Yes ma'am."

Hard as it was, Liz was adamant not to put Cody on psych meds again. From what she had seen, it confused the situation even more.

Liz handed the specialist the single-page spreadsheet she had prepared.

"These are his *Streptococcus pneumoniae* titer results," the doctor said. "PANDAS is believed to be triggered by *Streptococcus pyogenes*."

"Yes ma'am, I realize that. But may I please show you something?"

Liz handed her a copy of the parent comments she had collected from Facebook the day before. "I know this isn't an official study, but isn't it curious that all these PANDAS moms report tons of ear infections and pneumonia before their kids got the strep infections that drove them mad? Perhaps there's some connection? The onset may not just be related to throat infections—to group A strep."

Liz wanted to give this doctor all the information she thought might be pertinent for her to know, hoping she could see how the different pieces of this puzzle fit together.

"Maybe the high thyroid antibodies have something to do with this too?"

The doctor stared at the labs. "I honestly do not know."

To Liz, the spark of interest that she saw in the doctor's eyes felt like she had handed the doctor a puzzle piece she herself had not known was missing from her pile.

"I'll give you guys antibiotics to prevent strep for as long as you need them."

Liz could not stop her tears. Duke took insurance, and Liz was out tens of thousands of dollars taking Cody to all of the PANDAS specialists.

THE MANY HATS OF A PANDAS PARENT

During the consultation, Carol had asked the doctor whether PANDAS was reversible. After hearing the doctor say that it was not believed to be reversible, Cody was very upset, so he bolted. The nurse took it upon herself to call security for help. It took an hour before they found him.

"Whew, we could have done without all that!" Liz sighed, "The more people try to catch or restrain Cody—especially anyone who looks like an officer—the worse it gets. Instead, when he gets triggered, he needs space to sort things out in his head."

"What I've learned," Liz said as they got back on the freeway to head home, "is that to be a good mother to Cody, I have to wear many hats—that of a teacher, psychologist, psychiatrist, medical specialist, researcher, nutritionist, lawyer, warden, nurturer, financial provider, spiritual leader, insurance expert, alarm installer, IT expert, *and* a bouncer. I consider myself pretty capable, but this is ridiculous. I'd much prefer one job title. I'd love to simply concentrate on being a good mother."

It had been an exhausting trip, but the diagnosis from an institution on par with Vanderbilt and the antibiotics Cody got were well worth it.

HURTING ON MANY LEVELS

After they unpacked the car, Liz went to Cody's room and cracked open the door. "How are you feeling?"

"I don't want to talk about it."

Liz sat beside him on the bed. She held him tightly. Her son was hurting on so many levels. He laid his head against her chest as the tears streamed down both their faces.

"Cody, I promise you with all that I am: I will figure this out, one way or another."

This PANDAS mom was tired. But she was nowhere ready to take off her *researcher* hat.

CHAPTER 17

Contagious—or Not?

THE HONESTY OF AN OLD FRIEND

"Girlfriend, *what* is going on with you? You're wasting away!"

Liz's friend Trina had not seen her in years, so when those were the first words that came out of her mouth when she walked into the spa, Liz took her friend's concern seriously.

On her way home, she stopped by a walk-in clinic to see a doctor.

CHECKING TO SEE IF LIZ IS A CARRIER

Although her CRPS had calmed down with treatment, other symptoms were popping up. Liz began to wonder if her symptoms—like those of her children—could be related to an underlying infection. Liz opted to pay out of pocket so that she would be able to get the tests she needed while avoiding insurance hurdles.

"What seems to be the problem?" a male nurse asked as he entered the exam room.

"Well, I've lost about twenty pounds, and my friends are concerned."

"Are you on any medications?"

"No, I'm not taking anything right now.[27] But I have CRPS that I've ignored to focus on my son who's been very sick."

Liz chose her words carefully. If she said she was stressed out, they would blame everything on stress. Truthfully, she was under tremendous pressure, but less so than when the courts were involved.

"The CRPS seems to have stopped spreading when I started getting medical treatment and exercised regularly," she explained. "It might be that the CRPS may be spreading again."

She listed the symptoms she had experienced in the past six weeks. "First, I experienced chills for ten days, but I had no fever. Next, my neck got so tense that it scared me. And then my jaw got ridiculously stiff. But about two days after that, the rigidness subsided, and the tightness settled to the right side of my neck, jaw, and behind my ear. Also, my hair has started falling out again."

The nurse took notes as Liz kept talking. "Since then, a lymph node has popped up in my neck. I also feel a hard knot behind my earlobe and my jaw seems crooked. I went to the chiropractor to be adjusted, but the next day it was as if I hadn't gone at all."

Liz added, "Oh, and my son has a strain of *Streptococcus pneumoniae*, so it may help to do a titer test on me, just to be sure. Could you do a thyroid antibody test too, please?"

A few minutes later, the doctor entered the room and reviewed her chart. "Well, no offense to chiropractors, but they always say

---

27 **A note from the author:** To free up money for Cody's treatments, I had stopped taking all the medications my doctors had prescribed. My wrist had locked up again, but I could handle that. I did not mention it to the nurse, of course. It would have confused him further.

the vertebrae are out of alignment. But with the hair loss and weight loss," she smiled, "we do need to check your thyroid."

"It probably won't be a bad idea to check my thyroid antibodies. Can you also please do the *Streptococcus pneumoniae* titer test?"

"Well, we don't do that test here."

Liz handed her the details of a lab she knew ran those tests.

"I'll run a few tests here," the doctor continued as if she hadn't heard Liz. The technician came in to draw her blood.

CONTAGIOUS? OR NOT?

"In cases like yours," the doctor explained after the in-house test results were ready, "I listen if the patient is under stress, which I didn't hear that you were."

The doctor ran through the list of tests they had done and the results of those. No lymphoma. No elevated white blood count. No mono. "I've sent your thyroid hormone test to the lab. We'll have the results in a few days. In the meantime, I recommend you go see your primary care physician regarding the weight loss."

"Just to be clear, whatever I have is not contagious, right? I work closely with clients and I don't want the Centers for Disease Control and Prevention busting down my door because of some mutant strain traced back to me!"[28]

The doctor assured Liz that she had was indeed *not* contagious.

Once she got home, Liz jumped back into research mode, learning how easily many types of pneumonia—viral, fungal, *and* bacterial—could be spread. Since the doctor at the walk-in clinic

---

28 **A note from the author:** I was skeptical about this doctor's opinion as she shared that she had an enlarged lymph node that she ignored. The doctor was eventually diagnosed with Graves' disease, but she did not want to take the required medications and chose to have her thyroid removed. Hence, when she told me that I had wasn't contagious, I wasn't quite ready to take her at her word.

would not do a *Streptococcus pneumoniae* titer test, Liz could not be sure if that could be part of why she was exhibiting strange symptoms.

There were too many strange symptoms popping up around her for whatever it was making them all sick not to be contagious. Of that, Liz was convinced.

She scheduled an appointment with her primary care physician, so he could refer her to an infectious disease doctor.

While she had been focused on piecing together the puzzle to see what was wrong with Cody, Liz had not been working on clients at the spa. To be safe, she chose to continue keeping her distance.

CHAPTER 18
Side Effects

IT'S COMPLICATED

It was hard for Liz to believe a disease could be this complicated. The most recent PANDAS conference included a wide range of practitioners: immunologists, rheumatologists, neurologists, child psychiatrists, psychologists, educational psychologists, social workers, folks from integrative medicine, some from functional medicine, infectious disease specialists, and neurobiologists.

Liz had personally consulted with practitioners from nearly every one of these specialties about Cody.

What disease requires so much management yet remains completely unmanageable? And where are the pediatricians, pulmonary specialists, and ENTs?

THE IMPACT OF UNTREATED DISEASE ON FAMILY LIFE

Meanwhile, Liz started seeing a positive impact from Cody being put back on antibiotics prescribed by the doctor at Duke. It was not Levaquin, but it helped. He and Adam played well together. It was unbelievable to Liz what a difference this made to the family as a whole.

As she watched her sons play, she contemplated the fact that just perhaps, untreated infections could be contributing to the decline of the family in America. It certainly seemed to be the case with their family, and Liz knew many other families who were struggling in one way or another with various medical disorders. Her case may be extreme, but it was not isolated.

SUING THE COUNTY

After dinner one evening, Liz received a phone call from her lawyer, Connie. Connie had been Liz's guardian angel. She had saved them from the clutches of Judge Guffee and Melinda Ledford. Liz had decided to pursue legal action against the county.[29]

"You know that you are the only reason I am still able to continue, right?" Liz reminded Connie. "If I had lost custody of Cody, I wouldn't have been able to go on." Her eyes welled up.

"I'm just glad you've got Cody back," Connie assured Liz. She brought Liz up to speed on details for the lawsuit they had filed the previous week. The suit was against the county for their treatment of Cody while he was in their custody.[30]

"I sure hope that this changes things for the next child who comes through this awful juvenile court system."

"Me too," Connie assured her.

Recalling the events infuriated Liz. "When this all started, the police told me that I had to sign those petitions for runaway

---

29   **A note from the author:** Filing a lawsuit against the state wasn't about the money. It was about the responsibility that had been placed on her shoulders to do everything in her power to protect not only Cody but also the next child with PANDAS who may come through that courtroom. If they did not want to learn about it then, they sure were going to now.

30   To protect Cody, details of the trauma are being withheld.

and assault for them to help me find him. And then later, they turned around and said it was *my* fault because he had accrued so many petitions while Cody was in my care! I have to let the other mothers know what happens to their children when they ask the police or the court system for help."

Connie agreed. "Hey, I know you are already doing everything humanly possible to make sure this doesn't happen again by going to a lot of specialists," she said, "but I know you are looking very hard for a local doctor who's willing to learn about PANDAS and support Cody. I may have someone for you."

"You're so good to me," Liz said as she took down the details. The reality of a lawyer referring her to a doctor settled in as tears streamed down her cheeks.

Oh, God, what are we infected with that can cause such destruction, confusion, and division? Please show me, please guide me. You are the only one who knows.

CHAPTER 19

Yellow Butterfly

DESPERATE TIMES CALL FOR DESPERATE MEASURES

That night, Liz had a hard time sleeping. The reality of all she was trying to tackle took over.

How could I possibly solve this complex disease while also trying to turn the juvenile court system in America around? I'm only one person. One bite at a time.

On her way to the spa the next morning, Liz made an appointment with the doctor Connie had recommended. She must have clued him in on the severity of the situation, and he was able to fit Cody in later that same day.

Liz got halfway through an article on how bacteria could invade muscles when her client, Meredith, arrived for her appointment. As Liz led her to the treatment room, Meredith asked how Cody was doing. "You won't believe it, but he is pretty well. He did better on Levaquin, of all things, but that's a little tough to get, for some reason," Liz said.

Meredith told her that she used to be a rep for a pharmaceutical company that sold that antibiotic.

"Seriously?" Do you have any leftovers in a closet somewhere?" Liz half-joked.

"No, but you can order it online."

"Online?" Liz was stunned. "Don't you need a prescription?"

"Some countries with socialized medicine can ship it here without one."

What if it's not safe?

Liz had used a foreign manufacturer for her skincare line, and the suppliers she had worked with were sticklers about cleanliness and organic ingredients.

It seems like a feasible option—definitely something to look into.

SEEING THE DOCTOR WHOM THE LAWYER RECOMMENDED

This doctor listened intently as Liz went through the whole story of the *Streptococcus pneumoniae* titers, PANDAS, 19A, and Levaquin. In conclusion, Liz asked so to have some labs ordered to see if the Levaquin had killed the 19A.

"Sure, I need to look through these records a little more, though," he responded. "I'm not going to just order labs for the sake of ordering them. And you know the ones you are asking for aren't like the walk-in labs you can just run up the street and get."

Walk-in labs?

Liz made a mental note to find one immediately.

"We need to address Cody's vitamin D deficiency," he continued as he studied the spreadsheet with lab results. "And oh man, was his iron low for a while! How did you guys get it back up so quickly?"

"The only thing we have done was to treat him with antibiotics, so any changes could only be attributed to that. And his vitamin D hasn't been on my radar."

Liz had been as patient as she could be. "Could I be right about 19A causing PANDAS? I know there are a lot of numbers here, and I know my spreadsheets can be overwhelming, but could I be right?"

"When Connie told me about you, I visited your website and read your bio. You have a degree in biology; you developed your own treatment machine, and you helped formulate your own skincare line, so you seem to know your stuff," he said. "Send me an email with the labs you need, and we'll see what we can do."

Liz liked this doctor, but she did not get the sense that he could add anything significant. She was grateful to learn about walk-in labs, though.

If I could order labs and antibiotics on my own, we may be getting somewhere! Have I just been handed a do-it-yourself manual?

SOMEONE'S GOT TO KNOW HOW TO TREAT THIS

Liz was feeling more empowered and less reliant on the doctors she had lined up. Still, she was convinced that if she could get Cody's labs and his medical history in front of enough doctors, someone would be able to help her figure out where this infection has gone so they could get it treated.

She took Cody to see a pediatrician who earned her degree in psychology from Duke before going to medical school at Vanderbilt. "She may offer us the best of both worlds," she told her son.

"I've never heard of PANDAS being triggered by sinus infections," the pediatrician mused as she studied the abbreviated spreadsheet from Liz. "But it certainly looks like that may be the case for Cody."

Liz briefed her further. "The ENT found no bacterial colonies nor any hidden infections, but I'm convinced they're in his sinuses, don't you think? The immunologist marked Cody's immune system as fine. His lungs checked out great. The geneticist said his genes are good too. Both neurologists said he had nothing wrong other than bilateral maxillary sinus disease in 2010 and something in his ethmoid sinuses that wouldn't clear in 2013."

She continued, "We saw a doctor of Infectious Diseases at Vanderbilt, but he shut me down, so I don't want to go back. And he doesn't have any true psychiatric disorders; he doesn't have the genes for any. Behavioral changes that last six weeks or more can be considered a behavioral disorder, but Cody's go up and down."

The doctor looked in Cody's throat. "Gosh, it's beet red! Let me swab for strep."

"If a pathogenic strain of strep pneumonia is left untreated, couldn't that be what activated Cody's thyroid antibodies—or for that matter, activated other antibodies we haven't checked yet? The lining of the ears, nose, and throat are all connected, right? And the thyroid is next to the lining of the throat. Could this be what's causing autoimmune thyroid diseases?"

"Well, it's possible. It certainly could be causing some of them," the doctor replied before revealing that the strep test was negative.

"Listen, guys, I'm going to need some help here," she admitted. "Let's get an appointment at the Vanderbilt Pediatric Infectious Diseases Clinic with a different doctor."[31]

---

31 After the pediatrician had put in a referral with Vanderbilt Pediatric Infectious Diseases Clinic, the doctor who had seen Cody before called. They wouldn't allow Cody to see a different doctor.

REMEMBERING GOD'S PROMISES

"Mom, do you actually believe that I am going to be okay?" Cody asked on the way home.

"I know this is a hard road," Liz said, "but the day I brought you home from the hospital, the most beautiful, bright yellow butterfly landed right on your plump little arm and stayed for quite some time."

Cody was older now and tired of her stories, but he still enjoyed this one. Liz continued, "A butterfly represents new life, and I believe that was one of God's promises to you. With all my heart, I know that your story will help thousands of people. I don't know how yet, but I'm sure it will."

CHAPTER 20

Seeing the Bigger Picture

MAKING A SIGNIFICANT DISCOVERY

Once the children had gone to bed, Liz tried to relax and watch TV, but she could not shake the feeling that she was missing something. She had seen that group A strep was a major trigger for Cody's flares and felt certain that streptococcal pneumonia was a possible underlying contributor.

But why is his throat beet red?

The only thing Liz had not looked into thoroughly was mycoplasma.

Where does mycoplasma fit in? It first showed up in Cody's labs around the time baby Zach died and it seems to be playing a role somehow. In this puzzle, several pieces have fallen into place. But I still cannot see the bigger picture.

Liz was determined to figure it out.

Mycoplasma pneumoniae, she learned, was what caused so-called "walking pneumonia." What's more, the mycoplasma bacteria lacked a cell wall, which made them resistant to certain antibiotics. They could be parasitic in humans.

How can bacteria be a parasite?

Liz kept searching, but there just was not much substance to what she was finding.

I cannot find any current research on this organism. India has some research… and here's an article out of China. Wait, here's something that looks pretty thorough by someone at the University of Alabama at Birmingham from 2004.

The sixty-page research paper was way over Liz's head. She got out her notepad and pen and one at a time, she looked up the words she did not know.

It is what it is, and it's all that I have, so I'll just have to get through it.

After deciphering the scientific language, Liz started putting the ideas together again. What she found was shocking.

Mycoplasma is an intracellular organism—it can get inside cells. And like parasites, this organism took nutrients from host cells.

That mycoplasma could be feeding on Cody's vitamins and minerals infuriated Liz.

Mycoplasma fled from threats—other bacteria, viruses, even hormones, and chemicals—digging deeper into the body and its cells.[32]

Could that be why being exposed to viruses was so dangerous for Cody? I thought it was the "psych flu" caused by streptococcal pneumonia.

---

32 The scientific term for this phenomenon, whereby organisms direct their movements in response to certain chemicals, is chemotaxis. If pathogenic mycoplasma is inside the cells, introducing certain foods or hormones—especially cortisol, the stress hormone—it will cause the mycoplasma to burrow deeper into the tissues. The same is true when other infections that may be more virulent and are harmful to the mycoplasma's survival get into the bloodstream. However, once the mycoplasma is treated correctly, these things are not nearly as much of a problem.

But maybe it's the viruses causing the mycoplasma to burrow deeper into the part of the brain that controls neuropsychiatric symptoms?

Various other allergens such as red dyes, gluten, and hormones in dairy could cause it to flee and thus cause problems.

Mycoplasma was beginning to look like a major player in many horrible diseases.[33] In her research, Liz found countless species of mycoplasma, each with their own list of strains.[34]

It must have been divine intervention that she had done the research in the order she had because mycoplasma was turning out to give Liz an understanding of the bigger picture.

She started making connections between this organism not only to Cody's disease but also to hers.

TRYING TO GET TESTED

Liz was determined to have the author of this paper test her family. She clicked around until she found his number. "Umm, yes sir, I need to schedule an appointment to have my family tested for mycoplasma."

She told him where they lived and assured him that they would travel to wherever he was, explaining, "My son has this horrible autoimmune disease, and all these other weird things are going on with me and my children. I have a feeling that if mycoplasma is the root, and if we don't treat it in all of us, this hell will never end."

He stopped her before she could go any further, "If you think you have a mycoplasma infection, you can go to the Infectious Disease Department at Vanderbilt."

---

33 As the mycoplasma enters through the host cell membrane, it leaves its antigens on the surface of the host cells. This causes the body to create "confused" antibodies which, once created, will always recognize the hybrid host cell proteins as foreign and launch an attack. Antibodies cannot be destroyed. This causes autoimmunity.

34 For more information on these findings, visit our website. (Details at the end of this book.)

"Oh, okay," Liz said before hanging up.

Something feels off—very off.

TRUSTING HER INTUITION

Liz had learned not to ignore her intuition, and she had a new idea, so she called the Infectious Diseases Department at Vanderbilt. While she had worn out the doctors at Vanderbilt, she had not thought to contact researchers.

"Yes, hello, I need to speak with the expert on intracellular organisms."

"What?" the voice on the other end of the phone asked.

She was stumbling all over her words, "I'm doing some research and I need to speak with whomever has done any work on intracellular organisms or *Mycoplasma pneumoniae.*"

"We have someone who does work with *Chlamydia pneumoniae.*" Liz did a brief search and found that this organism could also be intracellular.

"Yeah, sure!" With that, Liz was transferred.

"Can I help you?" There was a professor on the other end of the line.

"I sure hope so!" Liz said excitedly. "I understand you work with the intracellular organism *Chlamydia pneumoniae.*"

"Yes, I do," he replied.

Liz launched in, "Okay, well, is it anything like mycoplasma? It sounds like they both can infect our cells and ultimately our tissue. I have a lot of questions, and I also need to get my family tested."

The professor paused, "There is only one man in the country that I know of who does any work on mycoplasma."

Silence.

"Umm, okay. Who?"

"Dr. Garth Nicolson out in California," he said.

Liz was typing the name in the search bar as he spoke.

PIECES OF THE PUZZLE ARE FALLING INTO PLACE

Wikipedia revealed that Garth L. Nicolson, Ph.D. is an American biochemist who made a landmark scientific model for cell membrane, known as the Fluid Mosaic Model.

Wow, I remember studying that in cell biology! This is the guy who figured that out?

She found Dr. Nicolson's website. His work covered cancer cell biology research, autoimmune illness, infectious disease research, and bioterrorism.

What in the world?!

Both fascinated and astounded, Liz read one research paper after another. The research confirmed what she was coming to believe as a significant piece of the puzzle concerning her family. It also expounded on her theories.

Liz had found *the* mycoplasma expert.

Dr. Nicolson had discovered the *incognitus* strain of *Mycoplasma fermentans*. The once benign organism had been genetically altered to be more harmful, to cause more severe symptoms, to be more immunosuppressive, to be more resistant to antibiotics, and to withstand very high temperatures.[35]

---

35 Dr. Nicolson identified the causal pathogen as *Mycoplasma fermentans*, which was a different strain from the natural pathogen, raising the possibility that it was a man-made biological weapon. This could be described as the mother of all genetically modified organisms (GMOs). Nicolson's written testimony to the US Senate in 1998 states: "We consider it quite likely that many of the Desert Storm veterans suffering from the GWI signs and symptoms may have been exposed to chemical/ biological toxins (exogenous or endogenous sources of these agents) containing slowly proliferating microorganisms (Mycoplasma, Brucella, Coxiella), and such infections, although not usually fatal, can produce various chronic signs and symptoms long after exposure." For a link to the research, please refer to www. whatswrongwellness.com.

Fevers could not even kill this? Someone made a weaponized *version of this organism?!*

Even worse, the genes from other debilitating viruses were woven into the genome of this pathogen. There were three prevalent bacteria. One contained the Epstein-Barr virus (which causes mono), another contained HHV-6 (a strain of herpes), and the third contained parts of the human immunodeficiency virus (HIV).

It's all tied together… Is that why Cody's HHV-6 was so high? I wonder which of these strains we have? Everyone's symptoms look different, this says…

Is it the version of mycoplasma that makes this so difficult to solve, or is it the pre-existing coinfections that muddy the waters?

That would make it nearly impossible to know what to look for, much less how to treat this. Is this how they intended it to play out? Brilliant criminals!

Liz kept reading Dr. Nicolson's findings and considered that there could be two pathogens—*Streptococcus pneumoniae* and mycoplasma—that could be suspects in the development of PANS/PANDAS.

Things began to make a lot more sense. Like criminals in cahoots, if two infections lived in the same host, then they could exchange their genetic information. This could explain how the traits of weaponized mycoplasma could end up spreading to other organisms within that host.

She also learned that pathogenic mycoplasma and other infections can be found in patients with amyotrophic lateral sclerosis (ALS), multiple sclerosis, Alzheimer's, Parkinson's, autism, chronic fatigue syndrome, fibromyalgia, and Gulf War syndrome. The gravity of the situation was dawning on Liz.

This is well beyond a super superbug. Is my family infected with a bioweapon?!

Liz was devastated.

How could we have gotten this? Mycoplasma isn't supposed to be this big of a deal! Where can I take my children to be treated? Who would know how to treat something like that?

She looked to see if Dr. Nicolson had any suggestions for treatment and was relieved to find a treatment protocol.

The protocol used phrases like *Herxheimer reaction*—the body's negative response to toxins released by bacteria when they are killed by medical treatment.

Light bulbs were coming on left, right, and center. More pieces of the puzzle were falling into place.

That's why Cody became exhausted when taking antibiotics and got worse before he got better. His body was having the kind of negative response to the organisms dying inside his body.

To push through and try to kill the mutant mycoplasma along with the other infections that had been collected over the years, Dr. Nicolson's protocol suggested antibiotic therapy for *at least a year*, possibly more.

STARTING TO SEE CLEARLY

The next profound insight was that psych drugs suppress the immune system.

No wonder people think they are getting better! It provides temporary relief but doesn't address the real issue.

Liz dug further into chronic fatigue syndrome.

Could this be what John had? Could it be that some of what drove John and me apart—rooted in the fact that he was chronically tired and depressed?—was also linked to mycoplasma?

The more Liz read, the angrier she got that more information was not available on this bacterium and the havoc it was wreaking throughout the country.

After hours of reading one research paper after another published by Dr. Nicolson, she called him and shared that her family may be affected by mycoplasma. "I'd like to schedule an appointment with you to come out for testing and treatment," Liz said.

But Dr. Nicolson was not a medical doctor, so he did not treat patients. He was a researcher and a professor. Unfortunately, he did not have any recommendations for a doctor close to Nashville who could treat them.

NOT EVEN PETS MISS OUT ON THIS

Not deterred by this minor disappointment, Liz continued her research. She read Dr. Nicolson's findings of how animals can contract this infection from their owners.

Buzz had been sick. If he had caught this from Cody, the mycoplasma would still be there.

Though Buzz got better on canine antibiotics, he was not himself and had strange symptoms he had not had before. He was shedding much more, had problems urinating, and his pupils were permanently dilated.

Plus, he would sometimes tear through the house like a mad dog, and he had abdominal tics that would last several minutes.

Liz called Buzz's veterinarian and asked for him to run a polymerase chain reaction (PCR) test—the test Dr. Nicolson recommended—on Cody's dog.

The veterinarian got back to her the minute the results were in.

If only our doctor's visits could have been that simple.

She pulled into her parking spot at the spa at the same time as her employees Donna and Belinda returned from their lunch break. She leaped out of her car. "I think I found the cause! Dr. Nicolson was right! And Buzz has it too!"

Knowing how many years Liz had been searching for what was making Cody sick, Donna and Belinda joined Liz in jumping for joy right in the middle of the parking lot.

Liz finally knew what to do for Cody—and for her entire family.

CHAPTER 21
Connecting the Pieces of the Puzzle

LIZ FINALLY PUTS IT TOGETHER

Liz had seen antibiotics work temporarily for Cody but had not tried them for herself. She did not want to order antibiotics from other countries, but she had done everything possible to get them in the States, so she ordered Zithromax, Doxycycline, and Levaquin from India.

If Buzz had this airborne pathogenic mycoplasma, surely, I do as well. Maybe this is why Cody got sick so quickly after stopping antibiotics. Maybe I am constantly exposing him.

Liz realized this was not her fault, but deep inside, she was riddled with guilt. If *she* were one of the reasons Cody kept getting sick, she would fix that. She would follow Dr. Nicolson's protocol for herself.

She took her first dose of antibiotics the week before Thanksgiving and waited.

By the end of the next day, her jaw and neck loosened. By day three, Liz was feeling better and found her words more easily, but her muscles ached, and her feet throbbed.

The next day, she was thrilled to find that she could bend her wrist again. After months of being locked, it had completely unlocked. At night, the location of previous knee injuries from years before burned intensely.

It was surreal.

THE SIDE EFFECTS OF HEALING

By day four, Liz's throat felt swollen. She noticed a black, pea-sized spot on the back of her throat. Her jaw ached and tingled.

Is this what was making my neck so tight and making me grind my teeth?

Meanwhile, she continued plowing through Dr. Nicolson's research. He wrote about his success healing his wife, Marie—a researcher at Baylor University at the time—who had nearly died from a mysterious disease he discovered was caused by mycoplasma.

A few years later, their daughter returned from the Gulf War with some of the same signs and symptoms her mom had shown when she was sick. Dr. Nicolson was able to make the connection between the Texas Prison Board, Baylor College of Medicine, and the Department of Defense.

Several attempts were made on his and Marie's lives, but they would not give up their relentless pursuit for truth. Unfortunately, Dr. Nicolson was ultimately chastised for recommending that veterans with PTSD and other chronic symptoms of Gulf War syndrome be treated with antibiotics.

Liz began questioning everything.

Was 19A the culprit? Or was the pathogenic mycoplasma the culprit? Which came first? If pathogenic mycoplasma was in the same host as 19A, it was a disaster. But just maybe what Dr. Pichichero had seen was pathogenic mycoplasma transferring its resistant gene to an already pathogenic 19A.

At this point, it did not matter which came first. All Liz knew was that she and her family would fight this. They would prevail.

HOW THE INFECTION SPREAD

As Liz worked through Dr. Nicolson's research, she was horrified to learn that experiments for the biological warfare agent used in the Gulf War were conducted in the Texas prison systems on death-row inmates. They had experimented with that population to observe the outcomes.

However, many of the other inmates not on death row started coming down with extraordinary, mysterious neurodegenerative conditions, as did some guards.

Wait! Steven had been in the Texas prison system!

Exorbitant rates of ALS cases, multiple sclerosis, and rheumatoid arthritis were recorded among the inmates and employees. The other prevalent infection identified in the Texas inmates and staff was MRSA.[36]

All of those boils we had! That must have been the cause of the staph infection Michelle got when she first came to live with us? And what about the fact that biological warfare experimentation was outlawed in 1972? How inhumane of the government scientists to use the prison systems as their laboratory! How could they not have considered that it could spread? One of the prisoners had to have been infected with mycoplasma pneumonia, which is airborne. How many weaponized organisms are out there by now?

---

36 Methicillin-resistant *Staphylococcus aureus* (MRSA) infection is caused by a type of staph bacteria that's become resistant to many of the antibiotics used to treat ordinary staph infections.

In the eighties, these illnesses crept into the local Texas community and beyond. These diseases that could be treated with antibiotics were ravaging lives everywhere.

Dr. Nicolson took his research to the senate in 1998. Why was this being kept secret?

LOOKING BACK

Liz read everything on mycoplasma she could get her hands on. She learned that it can be transferred with casual contact, but Dr. Nicolson's team thought it would take about twenty-four exposures to be infected. If someone was directly invaded by mycoplasma, that person would get extremely sick with flu-like symptoms that last seven to nine days.

I know exactly when and how this scourge was brought to our family, blowing us to smithereens. It started with the flu our entire family came down with when Steven first moved in. It entered our household as Steven stepped through the door, returning from rehab all those years ago. And it all started with those boils we got soon after.

Had we all contracted the weaponized mycoplasma from Steven?

REACHING OUT TO STEVEN

Liz knew with every fiber of her being that Dr. Nicolson's discoveries had played out in her family. To confirm it, she contacted her ex-brother-in-law. They had not spoken in years, but Liz still considered him a brother.

"When you went to that rehab center in Texas almost fifteen years ago," she launched the questions, "did you get sick with flu-like symptoms?"

"I sure did. How'd you know that?"

"Never mind that. What kind of medication did they give you?"

"Umm, a Z-pack—I think," he answered. "Why?"

The flu is a virus. You don't take antibiotics for a virus—only for a bacterial infection. But "they" knew damn well that what Steven and others were getting was not the flu. It was pathogenic Mycoplasma pneumoniae, *so they gave them Zithromax.*

"Were lots of prisoners transferred in and out of that facility?"

"Of course. But Liz, how do you know all this?"

"Just stay with me. Was it a year or so later that you started losing your hair?"

"Yes… Why?"

"How long after that did you learn you were HIV positive?"

"About three or four years later," Steven said.

"And nowadays, do you have muscle cramps, weight loss, trouble finding your words, and does it take a long time for you to heal?"

"Liz, please tell me how you know all that. You're freaking me out right now."

"How I know is not important, but you should know that mycoplasma has been thought to be one of the causes of HIV going into full-blown AIDS. You may want to ask your doctor for some Doxycycline so you can get a handle on the mycoplasma infection. If not, it'll end up killing you!"

"You know, I have been telling my HIV doctor and my neurologist that there's something else wrong with me other than HIV." Steven sounded defeated.

"Well, Steven, I am so very sorry that you are right."

TRACING BACK CODY'S PANDAS

We thought we were doing the right thing by letting Steven stay with us until he could get back on his feet, and now it's clear why his minor drug use turned into a major catastrophe. In the wake of

Steven's visit, our entire family was the sickest we had been in our lives.

It was hard not to be furious with Steven.

The reality of all that Liz was seeing started to sink in. Steven had reappeared a month or so before Cody had his acute onset of PANDAS!

"Dear God," Liz muttered under her breath, "what am I supposed to do with this information?"

After a few hours, her anger gave way to grief at the thought of all that her family—including Steven—had lost because of this organism.

Liz had promised Cody she would figure out what was wrong with him. But having finally done so did not feel nearly as good as she had dreamed of.

We weren't born to live our lives full of this much sickness and despair.

She could not believe all the proof she was gathering, so she wanted to see the patent for the organism. That night, she located the sixty-page patent and read it in its entirety.

The patent itself even implicates its role in chronic fatigue, Wegner's disease, Sarcoidosis Lupus as a causative agent or key cofactor.

The treatment recommended in the patent was Levaquin and Doxycycline.

It says right here that these diseases should be treated with antibiotics! None of my clients with Lupus or chronic fatigue have had antibiotics!

Maybe the doctors don't understand that it needs to be very long term and to rotate different antibiotics in with the other. With all of the ups and downs that came with Keflex, Biaxin, and Levaquin I sure have learned this the hard way.

LEAVING A TRAIL OF DEATH AND DESTRUCTION

Since Steven got out of rehab, he had lived with most of his family members at one time or another. In doing so, he had inadvertently left a trail of death and destruction behind him.

Could it be that much of his family's medical horrors were connected to them having been exposed to the weaponized mycoplasma?

His family's medical history since the time of his release included melanoma, thyroid disease, a brain malformation, suicides, rheumatoid arthritis, sarcoidosis, multiple other autoimmune diseases, heart problems, blood vessel inflammation, strokes, chronic fatigue, depression, addictions, CRPS, ovarian cancer, ADHD, ODD, PTSD, and PANS/PANDAS.

All this destruction occurred in Steven's wake, and he had no idea. How do I tell him? He and the rest of the family deserve to get better.

While the virulence may have lessened each time it was passed along to someone else, that did not make Liz feel any better. Although her brain told her it was not her fault that everyone around her had gone mad or become sick, her heart could not believe it.

It was overwhelming.

THE EFFECT OF PAIN MEDICINE

Over and over, Liz read all the studies and articles Dr. Nicolson had published and watched every lecture of his that she could find on YouTube. Among other things, she learned that pain medications suppress the immune system.

The nerve blocks that had worked for my CRPS were made up of steroids and pain medications. That's why they worked!

The same was true for psych medications—they also suppress the immune system. Everyone Liz knew with psych symptoms had eventually increased their medication to get better.

They were simply getting better at suppressing their symptoms. Those medications don't address the underlying cause, they simply hide the symptoms. Is this why we are hearing about so many immunosuppressant drugs being used now? Rituxan, IVIG, all those new biologics? This is their solution?

She also learned that sometimes, the children of infected parents could get better if they moved away. Their immune system could begin fighting, and many times without the constant re-exposure, they could recover. If they came back to visit for holidays or summer, they would be re-infected, and the cycle would start all over.

This is why John got so much better! He never would have gotten better had we stayed together.

Liz felt it important for her children to have a healthy and successful role model as a father.

John had to move out for him to get better, for all of us to recover.

Liz needed to make sure she was completely healthy so that she could help Cody for however long it would take for his brain to recover. She did not know where to begin, except to pray.

Life shouldn't have to be this difficult.

CHAPTER 22

A Simple Test

FOLLOWING PLAN B, FOR NOW

Liz had been ordering the antibiotics online, but now that she had spent over a hundred hours studying mycoplasma, she hoped she would be able to explain the situation better to her doctor. Despite her research and explanations, her doctor declined to order a PCR test or to give her antibiotics.

He did, however, send her for a mammogram for the swollen lymph nodes under her arm, and he agreed to put in a referral to an adult infectious diseases doctor at Vanderbilt.

MORE SIDE EFFECTS OF HEALING

Liz was wrecked by the die-off process. She could not move well and could not think straight, could not work. All that she wanted to do was curl up in a fetal position and sleep. But as a scientist at heart, she was also fascinated with what was happening. Although the backaches, night sweats, and intense sporadic itching that traveled from one place to another on her body were not comfortable, her anxiety and irritability were slowly fading.

Liz had never experienced anything like organisms dying off in her body before. As the dying organisms gave off toxins, it caused an adverse reaction. But she just wanted them all dead.

The relentless attack going on inside of me is not pleasant, but it has to happen.[37]

That night she lay awake digging at the front of her itchy thighs.

She looked down at the bruises that had appeared out of nowhere in the shape of a perfect circle around her kneecaps.

Well, I guess that injury eleven years ago wasn't runner's knee after all.

The black spot in the back of her throat was not nearly as concerning to her as it was for everyone else, but maybe that was her ticket to get the golden test.[38] The day after its appearance, she had a metal taste in her mouth, and all day, she smelled what seemed like stale cigarettes. It seemed that as the mycoplasma was dying, they released stored-up toxins.

She had only smoked for about a year, and that was four years earlier.

SEEING AN INFECTIOUS DISEASE DOCTOR

Liz's next appointment was with an adult infectious disease doctor at Vanderbilt, where she shared some of what she had learned from Dr. Nicolson's work.

---

37 **A note from the author:** With no guidance, this is what I believed at the time. Now we have ways to make this process much more manageable for clients.

38 The test referred to here is polymerase chain reaction (PCR) testing of nasopharyngeal aspirates.

This doctor took note of his name and book, *Project Day Lily*. Liz was encouraged by her interest.

She explained how much she had improved in the short time since starting the protocol. "I've gained three pounds, my heart rate is back down under a hundred, and my wrist moves after being locked for three years!"

Liz asked the doctor if she could please do a nasopharyngeal swab and a PCR test for *Mycoplasma pneumoniae*.

"What you're asking for is not traditional medicine," the doctor said as she laid her pen down. "I'll be happy to order you some blood tests, but the one you have requested isn't on our formulary. And if it's not on the formulary, I can't order it."

PCR tests are commonly used to diagnose infection. Why is the Mycoplasma pneumoniae *PCR test not on the formulary? Why is finding an infection not considered traditional medicine?*

"Well, you can't find it by doing a blood test, so I'd prefer to save my money," Liz replied.

"Okay, but let's take a look at that black spot."

Liz hopped onto the table. "Out of all the die-offs, this one is the most unique and obvious symptom."

"Did you ever smoke?" The doctor investigated the spot that would have been where the smoke hit the back of the throat while inhaling.

"Yes, for a little while; I'm ashamed to say."

"You should see an ENT," she said. "I'm so sorry that I couldn't do more for you after coming all the way down here. You're such a sweet girl."

Did she just call me sweet? I've been called many things in my life, but never sweet.

Liz certainly felt different. She felt more in control of herself. Whatever had been jerking her around for so many years was slowly powering down.

I guess that's what they were talking about during ADHD screenings when they asked if a child acted as if he was being driven by a motor.

The multiple TVs in her brain began powering down, one at a time. Viewing only two or three science channels at one time instead of ten or fifteen allowed her shoulders to relax a bit.

On her way back to the spa, Liz felt more confident than ever that her CRPS and other symptoms were the result of a *Mycoplasma pneumoniae* infection with a variety of unusual symptoms—something which doctors simply did not know about yet.

I know this is the honeymoon period of antibiotics and the worst is yet to come.[39] I also know that each antibiotic will bring about different die-off symptoms, but I needed to feel and see something working for me to truly believe this horrible story. Now, I believe it.

GIVING THANKS

That year, the children went to celebrate Thanksgiving with John and his new family. Liz decided to celebrate with her friend Anna and her family.

As she bowed her head for prayer, she felt immense gratitude for finding the answer to possibly end the anguish of more than five years.

---

39 Depending on the antibiotic used, the first few weeks can contain both die-off and also major relief in some people. Typically, true die-off starts anywhere from one to two weeks. There is no exact formula for these equations.

MAKING AN IRAQI CONNECTION

Liz got to the spa as quickly as she could and found her first client waiting. Rhonda was a tall, beautiful nurse who worked out religiously.

Liz could not help but notice her legs had purplish-blue veins unusually near the surface. Lots of clients had the beginnings of varicose veins and the like, but the fatty tissue in her thighs seemed irregular.

"Rhonda, when possible, you may want to ask your doctor about the congestion in your legs. Something isn't right."

"He said that very same thing! What, do you know something?"

"You're a nurse, so you'll understand."

Liz briefed Rhonda on the situation and explained the many other ailments that could be symptoms of this mysterious infection. Liz felt like she was constantly discovering new elements to this puzzle.

"Wow," Rhonda said. "Some of the things you mentioned sound like what my husband had when he came home from Iraq—and some of my problems."

"How long after your husband came home did you first start to get symptoms?"

"About six months."

That makes sense. Symptoms can take several months to develop enough to notice.

"And six months after that, I started losing my hair," Rhonda continued. "And I had an excruciatingly painful canker sore breakout. The doctor said he hadn't seen anything like it."

"Speaking of the military," Liz told her client, "Dr. Nicolson provided testimony to a House Committee that PTSD, chronic fatigue syndrome, fibromyalgia, Gulf War syndrome, and other chronic diseases are often caused—at least in part—by a bioweapon that was created called pathogenic mycoplasma."

Rhonda bolted upright on the treatment bed. "I believe him!"

Rhonda explained that she had also testified in front of the House Oversight Committee in 2007. "My husband was one of four private contractors killed in the streets of Fallujah by the Iraqis shortly before the first battle for control of the city."

"Oh, dear God, I am so sorry, Rhonda."

"It's okay, I'm dealing with it. But it's hard with all the unanswered questions that keep me up at night. My relatives all wanted to know what could have sparked such rage in locals to cause them to assault my husband and the other contractors' bodies like that," Rhonda explained.

"According to testimony, they were accompanying a convoy that was going to pick up kitchen catering equipment."

"Do you think the Iraqi insurgents may have believed that it was something other than kitchen equipment being carried on that convoy?" Liz asked tentatively.

"Yes, I do. It was really strange that all four contractors used for that mission had only recently been recruited. And they had to go in without the protection that had been specified in their contract."

Liz's eyes grew big as she continued the treatment. She began to wonder if Rhonda had contracted the original organism. She was getting in way too deep and wanted out. All she was trying to do was help Cody get better, but along the way, she kept stepping on landmines.

Liz did not scare easily, but this was a bit much—even for her. But she continued to listen as Rhonda explained even further.

On February 7, 2007, on her way into the hearing, she was surrounded by four armed operatives. Whether they were Black

Water or Secret Service, she never knew, but why the intimidation tactics?

Rhonda explained that later that same year she was relentlessly followed by unmarked vehicles. She owns a bail bond company, so when she had her officers run the tags and discovered they had been rented by the Department of Justice, she decided to stop asking so many questions.

What's the chance of this client—someone who has been coming to my spa for years— being the only person to be able to give me this information? This is no coincidence!

After several minutes of silence Liz said, "Well, we can never really know if biologicals were coming or going, blowing in the wind, or if your husband got sick from a preventative vaccine gone wrong. We were allied with Iraq in their war against Iran in 1980.

"Maybe Saddam Hussein ended up using it against us as well. Maybe those were the weapons of mass destruction President Bush felt so strongly were there. Honestly, I'm not trying to get into all of that because the truth is, we will never know. I just want people to get better. Let's focus on the future and get you back in shape!" Liz said, trying to remain in high spirits.

But truthfully, she was becoming increasingly nervous about her visit to the ENT's office. She had chosen one outside of the Vanderbilt system since she knew the test she needed was not on their formulary.

Hopefully, he will use Clongen Labs and give me a prescription for American antibiotics.

AT THE ENT OFFICE

The following day, Liz settled in the ENT's waiting room. She was reading Dr. Nicolson's book, *Project Day Lily,* to learn as much as she could about the history of what had happened to her family.

It was a difficult read, though, as Dr. Nicholson was an advanced molecular scientist.

Liz imagined writing a book someday in which she could share these hard concepts in a way more people could grasp them.

She looked up as a vet with a long beard helped his morbidly obese wife into a chair next to him before taking a seat himself. His wife laid her head against the back of the chair and placed a moist towel over her ear before falling asleep.

I wonder if she could be infected by 19A and mycoplasma...

Liz was moved to the exam room, but she kept thinking about the couple in the waiting room. She wished she could tell them that they should be tested for mycoplasma, that if they, too, were infected, that they could get better with antibiotics. But she knew they would never believe her.

The vets had been inundated with media on PTSD or other psychiatric labels and consequently, large numbers from their ranks ended up on psychiatric medications. The news was full of such stories.

"Good morning," the ENT entered the room. "I took a look at your intake."

Liz was quiet and patiently waited for the ENT to share his thoughts. After he looked at the black spot in her throat, Liz asked if he would biopsy the spot. She had learned that *Mycoplasma fermentans*[40] was very difficult to detect and was usually only able to be identified in necrosed tissue. She knew the black spot was probably just toxins, but what if...?

"Yes, I think that's a good idea."

---

40   *Mycoplasma fermentans* is a very small bacterium and is considered an opportunistic pathogen that is occasionally found in association with disease. However, due to its incredibly small size, the full extent of its role in human diseases is still under investigation. Like other mycoplasmas, it lacks a cell wall, which allows it to get into other cells.

"Would you please send the sample to Clongen Labs so they can test by PCR for *Mycoplasma pneumoniae* and *Mycoplasma fermentans?*"

If only he had seen what lengths I have been willing to go through to get the right test, he would agree!

"Well, I have a pathology lab that I generally use, and they do PCR testing."

Liz did not want to push, so she stayed quiet. But on the way out, she politely stated, "I'd prefer it if you used Clongen Labs, if possible."

To her surprise, the ENT called a couple of hours later, asking for the name of the lab she had recommended.

CODY STARTS THE PROTOCOL

Liz read Dr. Nicolson's protocol over and over and over again. As best as she could, she was committed to doing *exactly* as he said.

Once more antibiotics arrived, Cody joined Liz in following the protocol.

The die-off was fierce. But Liz wanted every mycoplasma infection, coinfection, opportunistic infection, burrowing spirochete, and virus out of their bodies.

Talk about a detox!

The more Liz thought about it, the simpler the concept seemed to her.

Of course, infections cause diseases! Why not? This theory would make psychiatric diseases the same as physical ones. They are all connected.

DIAGNOSIS CONFIRMED

A week before Christmas, after Liz had been on antibiotics for a month, she received a call from the ENT. Although they did not detect the ominous *Mycoplasma fermentans,* her test was positive for *Mycoplasma pneumoniae.* He agreed to prescribe her antibiotics for a year.

She was thrilled to have an official diagnosis, but she wasn't about to ask him for ten other kinds of antibiotics. She would fill the Doxycycline and cover the rest for herself.

This is a matter of life or death for Cody. I will not have a son in prison for the rest of his life. Not on my watch.

CHAPTER 23

The Cost of Getting Well

YET MORE SIDE EFFECTS

The effect of the mycoplasma dying off was brutal. Liz was shaking, sweating profusely, and getting uncontrollably angry about something minor that Cody had done.

Cody was also wild with rage.

It probably was the Levaquin that sent Cody into such a rage the night he cut his finger then broke his toe. Poor Cody!

She sank into a warm Epsom salt bath. It was all coming together in her mind.

TREATING MICHELLE AND ADAM

Liz printed the sixty-page patent, the protocol from Dr. Nicolson's website, both her and Buzz's positive results from Clongen Labs, and information on pathogenic mycoplasma to take to Dr. Brunner at Mission Clinic.

Buzz had been infected, so I have little doubt that Michelle and Adam are infected as well. They have different genetics and different infections from their childhoods, so they must be presenting differently.

"Thank you for meeting with me. I have some interesting information to share," Liz said as she handed Dr. Brunner the article on pathogenic mycoplasma.

She decided to withhold the hundred-page stack until she gauged his initial reaction. "Our dog and I both tested positive for *Mycoplasma pneumoniae*, and it showed up on Cody's labs as well. You have seen me in here with my children at least fifteen times over the years, and have you ever seen me or Cody exhibiting *any* symptoms of pneumonia?"

Kind yet firm, Liz continued, "No, because for over a decade, neither of us have had those symptoms. The mycoplasma shows up in *other* ways for us—through extrapulmonary symptoms. And now that we're on antibiotics, I've seen a *lot* of changes in both Cody and me. If Cody, our dog, *and* I have it, then Michelle and Adam likely also have it by now, and they'll need antibiotics so we can get rid of the infection."

As he skimmed the treatment protocol, he looked concerned. "Listen, I just don't want to see you chasing any rabbit trails for your family."

"Quite honestly, it feels like the last four years of my life have been nothing but rabbit trails. But this is no rabbit trail, Dr. Brunner, it's the end of the road."

Liz could feel the anger rising. "I'm not sure if you realize, but I have done *every single thing* you've asked of me for the last eight years. This time, I am asking that we go a different route, please."

"I owe you an apology if I haven't listened to you very well," Dr. Brunner said calmly, continuing in his usual line of questioning.

Adam isn't doing any better after adding the lunchtime dose of ADHD medication?"

"Not one single bit. Would you please give me a prescription for the antibiotics he and Michelle need?"

He reached for his prescription pad. "Let's get Adam psychoeducational testing."

Clearly, the apology for not listening was mere lip service. Grateful she had not hung her hat on Dr. Brunner for correct treatment, Liz decided that trying to convince doctors of this was a waste of time.

I'll just have to do the best I can and ask Dr. Nicolson questions when I can.

CAROL SEES THE DIFFERENCE

When Carol came over on Christmas morning, the children ran to hug her. She beamed. "Honey, I wouldn't have believed this if I didn't see it with my own eyes. The children seem different. And the only thing you've changed is giving antibiotics?"

"Well, that *and* I got rid of the ADHD meds—they weren't helping anyway. Mom, we have a long way to go, a tough row to hoe. And I have so much more to learn.

"From what I've learned, Cody will continue to flare until this organism is under control, and even after that, we have to deal with the autoimmune response. But I will not give up. The chaos and trauma have to end."

They sat on the same couch where the chaos began, the couch Cody had laid on to recover from his strep-turned-PANDAS-turned-hell four years earlier—almost to the day.

"Remember how you told me about your brain hurting? I think I know what caused that feeling," Liz began.

"I'm all ears."

"Working with vets with PTSD for years as a therapist put you at a much higher risk of catching something yourself," Liz explained. "Because—believe it or not—chronic fatigue and PTSD can be contagious."

"What? Those guys had been through traumatic experiences. How can PTSD be contagious?"

"Isn't it true that some of the vets with PTSD didn't even go to war?"

"Well, yes, but those vets had traumatic childhoods."

"Mom, think about it. Lots of people who have had traumatic childhoods don't snap like people with PTSD. Could it be possible that people who have suffered trauma and who *also* have this infection could have symptoms of PTSD?"

"I suppose..."

"If the trauma center of the brain is affected by an organism somehow, therapy alone cannot fix it."

"So, you're against therapy?"

"Of course not, but the infections have to be addressed as well."

"And psych meds? My clients have felt much better on antidepressants and the like," Carol pointed out.

"Yes, psych meds may make them feel better. But, in cases where an infection is present, the psych meds only suppress the immune system's *response* to the infection, allowing the patient to *appear* to be improving; but in reality, the disease is continuing to slowly move to other tissues, taking them over."

"Goodness!"

"It's simply a matter of time before other medical issues emerge, which may cause more psychological stress that could trigger trauma symptoms to return," Liz continued.

"Cody must recover *medically* if he is going to have a chance to recover from the *psychological* trauma from all he's been through over the last four years. Therapy cannot stop an infection from spreading. Unless we do something about the infection in the cases where an infection is present, vets are going to keep snapping, and school shooters will keep shooting."

"School shooters!?" Carol crossed her arms. "You can't possibly think that *everything* is the result of an infection."

"I'm not saying this causes *everything*, but you have to admit, it could at the least be playing a role in many cases."

Carol looked over at the children who were calmly, happily enjoying the Christmas festivities. She turned to Liz. "Do you think they could help me?"

Liz smiled. "I do." Liz hugged Carol tightly as the oven timer went off. "Let's go check on our Christmas dinner."

GOOD TIMES AND HARD TIMES

When the Harris family made it through the rest of the holiday season without incident, Liz felt that they had truly received a Christmas miracle.

But with financial strains and intense die-off symptoms, times were hard. Through the cramping, itching, bloating, and aching, Liz often reminded her children that they had been given the gift of knowledge. They could get through anything with the belief that it had an end.

A few weeks after Carol had started taking antibiotics, she called Liz with an update. "I feel really good, and I've even started looking for a new job. These antibiotics may be helping more than my psych meds."

Because Carol had continued her psych meds, her die-off wasn't as noticeable. Eventually, she would need to wean off those as well but for now, Liz was glad her mom was doing so well.

Liz hung up and headed to the high school to attend a meeting regarding Adam. As she drove down the winding country road leading to the school, she realized to her surprise that she was looking forward to learning their findings.

Adam's psychoeducational test results turned out to be just fine.

Liz left the school feeling even more confident about her conclusions, but also more overwhelmed. As she listened to all of the words being tossed around at Adam's evaluation, she began seeing everything from a different angle.

Societal shaming and negative labeling are never acceptable—this must stop.

LOOKING FOR A NEW HOME

Another project that could not wait was finding new housing. Liz was so far behind on her mortgage that the bank took her home. Her family seemed to be catching everything but a break. The medical and legal bills had been too much to overcome.

Everyone felt an enormous sense of loss at moving out of the home they had been in for six years. Cody struggled the most because he was leaving Rusty, who had been laid to rest in their backyard. Loss kept piling onto loss, but now was *not* the time to give up.

CHAPTER 24

Not Yet Quite to the Finish Line

UP AND DOWN

The Harris family drove around for the next two days searching for temporary housing. Due to their recent foreclosure, there was only one option. Fortunately, it was a nice apartment complex near downtown Franklin.

As soon as they were settled, Cody began weekly therapy sessions to process the trauma he suffered at the juvenile detention center. He was progressing well, and Cody desperately wanted to attend school, so Liz agreed to let him go back full time.

After only a few weeks, however, he flared.

"Psych symptoms," he texted Liz.

Cody's doing everything he's told to help him recover, but the first time he goes back to school full time he flares. Will he ever be able to be in groups again?!

These psychological symptoms quickly escalated, prompting the assistant principal to threaten him with in-school suspension (ISS). This punishment echoed his experience at the juvenile detention center—no talking, moving, or exiting the room was permitted.

The thought of possible confinement made Cody respond in an aggressively defiant manner.

Liz requested that Cody clean toilets or mow lawns instead—just not something that could trigger memories of his weeks in solitary confinement. She even brought in a letter from Cody's psychiatrist stating that being confined was dangerous for him, but the assistant principal would not budge.

The ISS was enforced.

Cody only made it through the first few hours of confinement. When the ISS teacher threatened another student with the cops, Cody darted out the door in a panic. He texted Liz, and she found him shaking with fear in the school parking lot.[41]

Something is going on besides PANDAS here. Is this the plus *Dr. T mentioned?*

THE IMPACT OF TRAUMA

Liz related the situation to Cody's new therapist. "He ran out of the school. He is defiant, angry, and is having nightmares."

"These are all symptoms of trauma," the therapist explained. "Sounds like Cody's PTSD must have been aggravated by the heavy hand of the administrator."

It turned out that the therapist was correct. On the symptom scales for PTSD, Cody scored a 36, more than double the score that qualifies an adolescent patient as having the disorder.

---

41 Damage to the brain caused by infections (e.g., meningitis and encephalitis), by tumors, and by metabolic disorders cannot be corrected through disciplining a child. In addition to treating the infection or disorder, behavioral shaping—not discipline—is needed.

Dr. T was also correct. Cody's PTSD was making his PANDAS worse.

To help reduce his symptoms of PTSD, Cody's new therapist tried eye-movement desensitization and reprocessing (EMDR) therapy. As a part of EMDR, a patient recounts the trauma experienced in detail.

This therapy backfired, though, and pushed Cody over the edge.

Maybe it was too much, too fast. Maybe Cody should not be going to any kind of therapy during a flare.

Liz watched helplessly as her son spiraled out of control. Cody said that he could not stay at home but could not explain why. And he refused to take his antibiotics.

Liz knew that the more she chased him, the farther he would run. He texted her occasionally as he stayed with his girlfriend or his grandmother, but Liz was worried sick and barely slept.

Something was terribly wrong.

While they were having a heated exchange, flashing lights lit up his bedroom and reflected off the mirror.[42]

No wonder he doesn't want to stay at home!

For the time being, though, the Harris family was stuck in that apartment.

REALIZING THE DANGER OF TRAUMA

Liz was finally able to get her son back on the antibiotics and was doing her best to manage the die-off. But she had not realized the effect PTSD could have on her son.

---

42 **A note from the author:** It was not obvious in the daylight. However, at night, sirens and flashing lights from the juvenile detention center and jail two blocks away came in through Cody's bedroom window, triggering his PTSD. For the time being, he had no safe space to retreat and relax, to heal and process in peace.

Cody was petrified of police officers, and the ISS had resurfaced those fears. In turn, the EMDR had made things even worse. Cody's PTSD was dramatically exacerbating his condition, and he was desperately trying to self-medicate with alcohol to soothe the feelings that it unearthed. Little did they realize that mycoplasma feeds on alcohol.

Liz spent the week following him from place to place trying to separate him from one beer after another. He simply would not give up drinking. Liz, meanwhile, would not give up trying to help her son.

Next, while intoxicated, Cody jumped in the golf cart owned by the complex and drove it around their apartment parking lot in broad daylight. He was charged with felony theft, along with possession and consumption of alcohol by a minor.

Even though there was no defense for joyriding, Liz explained to the officers that PTSD was a mental condition and begged them to change the call to one of a medical nature. They would make no allowances, though.

Luckily, they simply took him to the emergency room for evaluation and released him to her. It was bittersweet to drive her barely sober son home at three in the morning. She took him out of EMDR therapy indefinitely. To avoid future events, Liz would have to find a trauma therapist who was willing to learn about PANDAS.

Cody's flare was compounded by PTSD, EMDR, and alcohol, which had catapulted him into a dark and evil place.

Eleven days later, Cody began to come out of the flare.

Are flares the same thing as benders—when addicts take off for days on end? Maybe when alcoholics go off on benders, they are actually having flares.

Cody's autoimmune dissociation had improved slightly, though. He was no longer a completely different person who talked to her as if from another realm.

ADDRESSING CODY'S SUBSTANCE ABUSE

Several days later, Liz took Cody for a psychological assessment to address his substance abuse she had observed the prior weeks. Thinking the clinic director may recommend outpatient treatment, she was surprised when he walked out saying, "I'd like Cody to come once a week for group therapy."

"Based on what I saw last week, my son needs therapy once a *day*!" Liz suggested. But the director did not agree.

It was true that Cody looked and acted fine for the hour it took to assess him, though.

Liz felt horrible that she was unable to stop the cycle of triggers during flares, which led to self-medication and trouble.

If only we had been able to stop all this thirteen years ago, then he would not have ended up with PANDAS, he would not have landed in jail and solitary confinement, and he would not have PTSD!

Heading to the car after the assessment, she told Cody, "This is the most convoluted situation I could imagine. Something you must have been exposed to at school caused you to flare, and then during the flare, your PTSD was triggered, and you stopped taking your antibiotics and started drinking beer like it's soda! But it's not. Alcohol feeds mycoplasma. Meanwhile, your body's releasing stress hormones which adds more fuel to the fire—a recipe for disaster!"

"Mom, I don't even know what you're saying right now," Cody complained as he put on his seatbelt.

"We've only been doing this antibiotic therapy for a few months, son. We will just have to be vigilant when you're not in flares. We have a long way to go. We will have to deal with the trauma later. But we will get through this, one way or another."

Liz looked at Cody. "You do have Buzz. He's getting better too—he's shedding less and is much calmer. He has many healthy years ahead of him now that he's getting the right medical treatment."

Cody cracked a smile.

FROM IN-HOME DETENTION TO HOMESCHOOLING

Now that Cody had another in-home detention order in place, Liz had no room to discipline him on her own accord. The courts had taken everything away from him already. No bargaining chips remained.

Being confined to the apartment overlooking the detention center all day was not good for his mental health, though. Taking Cody to work with her was not good for Liz's mental health, but she had no choice.

"I guess we're stuck here or at the spa for a while," Liz said.

Cody groaned, looking defeated. "It's spring break!"

"I'm sorry, son," she responded. She felt as defeated as her son, if not more. In this multi-year battle, Liz had lost herself.

Do they want me to lose absolutely everything? I can't focus on my work—my only source of income—knowing that my child is either locked down in our apartment or stuck upstairs in the spa. And if he bolts for whatever reason, I will be going to jail along with him if I don't tattle. What the hell?

And on top of all this, there is no way I can send Cody to school in this state.

Just when it looked like things were turning around, Cody's PTSD was making his PANS/PANDAS worse again.

Liz was at her wit's end. While she had been advocating for Cody to get an IEP with a lessened workload and had hoped to manage his schooling at home while he got better, her intention was not to have Cody homebound 24/7—especially not while dealing with PTSD and substance abuse, none of which she felt equipped to deal with.

Liz had no choice but to pull her son out of school completely and to opt for homeschooling him—another thing she did not feel qualified to do.

To make things worse, Cody was fifteen by now and even more adept at slipping out than he was in his early teens.

What Liz wanted was for her son to get better. What she wanted for herself was some help in getting him to that point.

COULD THIS GO FASTER?

Dr. Nicolson's protocol would take more than a year. Liz tried desperately to figure out a way to get Cody better quicker than that.

Maybe I could figure out something that would kill the bacteria faster so the symptoms would be more manageable...

Common sense told her that the fewer bacteria in the cells, the less dramatic the response may be.

USING PSYCH MEDS TO MANAGE PSYCH SYMPTOMS

From her continued research, Liz learned more about intracellular infection. When the mycoplasma infected a host cell, they would leave proteins on the surface, and the infected person's immune system would see the mycoplasma proteins remaining on the host cell wall as enemies and attack them.

In the same way, strep bacteria caused the body to launch an autoimmune attack.

This was the root of autoimmune issues. Eventually, most cells die and, during treatment, are replaced with new ones. But it takes time for cellular turnover to take place.

We will just have to wait for his infected cells to turn over before this hell can pass. Unfortunately, neurons may take longer to regenerate. I must do something that can bring the virulence of these flares down until the infection is gone.

Liz called her psychiatrist for help. "Is there any way we can use the fact that psych meds suppress the immune response to our advantage? We need to keep Cody's psych symptoms under control until more of the infection is out of his system."

"Yes, but they have to be carefully managed, and it takes a while for them to be effective."

"Well, whatever it takes. Now that I understand what is happening, I know we have to suppress the immune response until more of the infection is under control."

We are back to square one, using the psych meds for the psych symptoms.

While it made Liz angry and uncomfortable to give her child medication with unknown long-term effects just to keep him out of the detention center, she knew this was a temporary solution.

Until they had completed Dr. Nicolson's protocol, the flares triggered by the mycoplasma would show up.

As for the trauma Cody had suffered at the hands of the state which led to his PTSD? It would take therapy, psych meds—but only for a season—and much patience.

In the end, it would be another two years before Cody would be healthy.

Through it all, Liz would not give up.

Her faith had carried her this far. Plus, she had been given hope that this would not last. And she had love. Without that, this puzzle would be unbearable.

CHAPTER 25

Helping Others

SUMMER 2020

"That was *so* much fun!" twenty-eight-year-old Kelsey burst through the front door ahead of the rest of the Harrises.

A beaming Liz followed Kelsey into the kitchen. "I love canoeing," she said for the umpteenth time that day, "especially with you four!"

"What are we going to grill?" Adam asked as he and Michelle filed in next.

"Salmon, I'm sure," Cody laughed as he closed the front door behind him.

Liz walked out to start the fire. Having all her children together and healthy was the best birthday gift.

DIFFERENT PUZZLE PICTURES FOR DIFFERENT PATIENTS

It had been a long and hard road—one that could have been avoided. Although Liz's primary focus was on helping her son and her family, it broke her heart to watch the others with PANDAS be stuck.

Despite doctors saying they would outgrow the flares, they did not. Many were institutionalized for life.

But Cody's puzzle turned out differently. He got well.

Liz was determined to help other families learn from the mistakes she had unknowingly made. Throughout her family's journey to healing, Liz was forced to search for answers, as well as follow her gut, trusting her intuition for what was right. But that should not have been the case.

She had learned a lot, seen a lot, and prayed a lot. She would use this experience to help guide other families.

In the process, Liz discovered that using nutraceuticals— foods containing health-giving additives and having medicinal benefits—could provide a safer way to help people heal.

She also gained knowledge about the right psych medication to use initially—something she would have given anything to have known ten years earlier!

CODY'S RECOVERY

For Cody, though, recovery had been a long, hard road. Much of it was due to a lack of guidance related to PANS/PANDAS. But recover he did—bit by bit.

It had been almost three years since he had the long, drawn-out flares of the past. Now that the cause had been addressed, Liz was able to find a medical professional who would give Cody a shot of Rocephin at any sign of an onset, preventing an attack on his brain by "confused" antibodies. This has saved them the relentless trips to the ER, psych wards, and jails.

RESISTANCE TO CHANGE

Liz knew it may take a while for the information about mycoplasma to get out and be widely embraced. But she and her team had such success with their clients; there was no denying their approach works.

And she knew that she was in good company when it comes to trying to convince the medical community of something they simply were not accustomed to.

In 1847, for example, a Hungarian doctor named Ignaz Semmelweis was the first one to inform the medical community that diseases were not spread by bad odors, but instead, through contaminated hands. He urged doctors to wash their hands, insisting that diseases were spreading from their hands to the instruments they were using and then to their patients. Because he could not prove his theory, they simply laughed at him.

When Louis Pasteur started publishing papers on germ theory nineteen years later, Semmelweis had been admitted to an asylum following a nervous breakdown. He died just as Pasteur started providing proof that the Hungarian had been right all along.

There was Dr. John Snow who, in 1855, had a difficult time convincing the medical community that cholera was being spread through contaminated water. He worked at proving his theory until he was successful.

And then, of course, there was Sigmund Freud whose ideas around talk therapy in the early twentieth century took many decades to permeate the world, but today, having a therapist is strongly encouraged and widely embraced.

No matter where or when, people still have a hard time considering there may be another explanation for the problems before them. It is easy to be stuck with what we have been taught, making it hard to consider a novel theory or explanation.

BACK TO THE SUMMER OF 2020

As Liz and her children sat down to enjoy their salmon, she reminded them, "One day, your grandchildren will be talking about the days when we did not believe that multiple chronic infections caused autoimmune diseases, when we refused to accept that psychiatric symptoms could be rooted in untreated infections, or that addiction could be a legitimate disease rather than simply a moral failure. I may not be alive to see it, but I'm convinced that day will come."

THE GREATER IMPACT OF GETTING WELL

"Buzz! Gus!" Cody called, and his dogs came charging down the stairs and out into the backyard with the family.

"Oh my gosh! I can't believe how big Gus is!" Michelle laughed as she hugged the Great Dane.

Still a puppy, Gus already weighed 120 pounds. "Can you imagine this guy when he's fully grown? He'll gain another sixty pounds! These two are *so* much fun to watch," Cody beamed.

He offered to show his siblings his new animal room after dinner. There, he kept several reptiles and some fish. Since Cody's pets were no longer affected by his former infection, he enjoyed adding to what he called his "farm."

It did not take long for the attention to shift to Liz's business. The kids were excited about how well the spas and the new wellness center were doing.

"I think it's awesome that you guys are helping so many people beat this," Kelsey said proudly.

Cody was considering joining the team at Liz's wellness business, determined to help kids and their families conquer PANS/PANDAS and other mycoplasma-related challenges.

"There's nothing like learning from someone who's gone through what you are going through," Liz assured them.[43]

She shared that Dr. Nicolson's most recent paper pointed out that the number one reason for treatment failure was not treating patients for long enough. Some people have been sick for so long, it may take a few years to get them turned around—especially to help them overcome the mindset that they are sick.

"It can be extremely challenging to turn that piece around. We must help keep people motivated to push through. Cody, that's where your life coaching can be the most valuable."

The others could not agree more. They all knew it may take a while for the information about mycoplasma to get out and be widely embraced.

EXPOSED TO THE CORONAVIRUS

Not long after this get-together, Cody woke up one morning with a fever of a hundred-and-four.

While others were concerned about the possibility that Cody had COVID-19, Liz saw the good in the situation. Before, being exposed to a new pathogen would trigger a flare. Now, Cody's immune system responded the way it should. It fought the virus and resulted in him having a fever. It was a perfectly normal reaction.

---

43 **A note from the author:** On the other side of the mycoplasma infection, Cody had his first fever of 103 since he was very young. Getting a fever is the body's innate immune response. Now, he got sick like a person without an autoimmune disease would get sick. There were very few psych symptoms—if any. It must have been a pathogen his immune system had never tried to fight in the past. However, due to the molecular mimicry, Cody's would have had psych symptoms if he would have contracted, group A strep, streptococcal pneumonia, mycoplasma, or any of the infections of his youth. Now, at the first sign of psych symptoms, Cody goes to get a shot of Rocephin.

One of the side effects of COVID-19 is multisystem inflammatory syndrome in children (MIS-C). Liz came to believe that the coronavirus likely triggered MIS-C in undiagnosed or mistreated PANDAS/PANS patients.

As for Cody, he recovered as well, just as most twenty-one-year-old males with COVID-19 did.

Cytokine storms had been something the Harris family had dealt with for over a decade. Liz found social distancing, the wearing of masks, and frequent hand washing recommended during the pandemic to be comforting. It could protect more children from pathogens—whether man-made or natural.

DESPERATION, TENACITY, AND VICTORY

"Desperation is the raw material of drastic change," William S. Burroughs once wrote.

In the years of trying to find what was wrong with Cody, with her, and with her family, Liz had experienced levels of desperation she had never been acquainted with. But she was more than just desperate, she was tenacious.

And after many years, she felt victorious. She even stumbled upon what may be wrong with a lot of the world!

Now that they were well, she was as determined as ever to share with others what she had learned. The quest had cost her marriage, her home, and even her sanity for a season. It had also cost her more than a million dollars to get to this point.

Liz had several years where all she thought about was a solution to their family's problems. The more she read and witnessed, the more she continued to put pieces of the puzzle together.

She learned that decades earlier, there was far more experimenting going on than what took place in the Texas prison systems in the 1980s.

As a result, Liz looked at her childhood from a different angle. She had several family members go through PCR testing, and they all tested positive for mycoplasma.

How they all got infected, they will never know. It does not matter.

There is a lot of speculation around the origin of weaponized mycoplasma. Was it an experiment gone wrong? Or was it a bioweapon?

The answer to that mystery does not matter either.

What matters is that there is a viable treatment.

The treatment is neither easy nor is it quick. But it works.

WHAT TO DO IF YOU NEED HELP

Years ago, Liz assured Cody that his story will help many others. She is still convinced of that, which is why she launched a wellness center to help other parents figure out much faster what could be wrong with their child.

Liz's wellness business focuses on finding the root of inflammation. It has been found that inflammation can do a lot of damage to neural pathways. This can impact thought patterns and wreak havoc not only on people's physical health but also on their mental and psychological health.

If you would like more information, please visit www.whatswrongwellness.com.

UPDATE

UPDATE ON THE HARRIS FAMILY

Once Cody completed the protocol, he was able to catch up on his education at a local community college. By the summer of 2020, he was one semester away from earning his associate degree and planned to continue his education with a focus on neuroscience.

He also earned a personal training certification from the National Academy of Sports Medicine. In addition, he earned several life coaching certificates, got his brown belt in jujitsu, won several tournaments, and he started doing jujitsu coaching on the side.

Cody also teaches guitar lessons and has joined the praise team at church.

Liz is currently working on a Master's in Molecular Medicine. She manages her spas and sees clients for the wellness center rather than fighting for custody, trying to solve a mysterious disease, and managing die-off symptoms.

The entire family had suffered because of Cody's PANS/PANDAS, but Liz found solace in knowing that they had the rest of their lives ahead as a healthy family. She knew there would still be ups and downs, but they would take things as they came.

After much hesitation initially, Kelsey finally started treatment, and within just a few months, her anger melted away. She turned into a loving young woman.

Each time Liz witnessed a transformation such as that, she realized just how detrimental untreated chronic infections can be to families.

Michelle was no longer exhibiting any signs of ADD and had completed an associate degree. She had transferred to Middle Tennessee State University where she would go on to earn her bachelor's degree in physics.

Adam was not convinced he needed antibiotics and nutraceuticals, nor was he convinced he needed to go to college. But he is happy, and for the time being, that is all that matters.

Unfortunately, Steven passed in his sleep at the age of forty-five. He had tried doxycycline for a few weeks but found the die-off to be unbearable.

UPDATE ON OTHER PERSONS IN THIS REAL-LIFE DRAMA

Colleagues who worked closely with Liz and had been affected by this organism completed the protocol. They are doing great.

Mark, however, is still very sick, and Karen has been diagnosed with schizophrenia.

Dr. Meneely "retired early." Liz ended up not filing a medical malpractice lawsuit against him.

Considering the extent of torture her son went through under the care of the county, Liz took the county to court, though. A panel of judges at the Sixth Circuit Court of Appeals granted qualified immunity to Steve McMahan, the supervisor responsible for the psychological torture of Cody at the detention center. They exempted him from all liability, after which he "retired early."

Judge Guffee got off scot-free due to absolute judicial immunity. At the time of publication, she still presides over the future of troubled youth in Williamson County.

In Tennessee, solitary confinement is still a legal practice in youth detention centers. Cody had been kept in solitary confinement twenty-three hours per day for weeks on end, at the time leading to him attempting suicide.

The Harris family is committed to continue speaking out against this type of state-sponsored psychological torture.

In the end, Cody ended up in the right hands—professionals who have come to believe in PANDAS and who have been truly supportive of the Harris family and this population as a whole.

Connie Reguli continues to work on behalf of other families suffering from the legal pitfalls of PANS/PANDAS/AE.

In Glynn Dilbeck, Cody finally had a safe place to start processing the abuse and medical trauma he had endured during his youth. Glynn is an extremely competent licensed senior psychological examiner and certified addictions therapist, among other qualifications. He was keen to learn about PANS/PANDAS.

After some time of working with Cody, Glynn was able to spot a flare coming on as well as Liz could. This is important since the transition from a non- or limited-functioning ability to functioning requires work on the patient's part and a competent therapist.

Cody also worked with Dr. Jason Tharpe from ChiroCore Wellness for neuro-biofeedback, which helps retrain faulty thought patterns. Dr. Tharpe was kind and truly cared about Cody. He was committed to helping him achieve full recovery.[44] None of this could have been nearly as effective without the right medical treatment beforehand.

---

44 In partnership with www.whatswrongwellness.com, neuro-biofeedback is now available remotely.

After having seen so many doctors, Liz finally found a brilliant and open-minded board-certified physician's assistant to help Cody. After having read an earlier version of Liz's research, he was able to put all of the pieces together and began recognizing these connections in his practice.

Not only did he look for the infection, he also figured out how to stop a flare at the onset. He has been able to prevent much devastation by treating psych symptoms with antibiotics. Through her wellness business, Liz has sent many patients his way whom he has been able to help before their PANS/PANDAS progressed as far as it had with Cody.

If you want more information about possible testing and treatment for you and your child, please visit www.whatswrongwellness.com.

ACKNOWLEDGMENTS

Through the darkness, there were those who shone like a bright light.

Dr. Sparks: Your role was pivotal. Thank you for believing in me when nobody else did. Thank you for being there during one of the scariest points in my life and for ordering the test that finally got us on the right path. And the deposition? You nailed it! Who knew you were a court expert too! God was watching out for us. Some people are just angels.

Connie Reguli: I can never thank you enough. You gave me my child back when no other attorney stood a chance. You learned AE like a rockstar and questioned the experts like you had worked with this diagnosis forever. You fight for the orphans and the poor like we are supposed to do. You are my inspiration to press on no matter the cost.

Dr. Trifilletti: Most doctors would not have touched our case with a ten-foot pole. You dismissed all of the chaos going on to focus on the root of my son's illness and through watching you sort and solve things the way that you did I was able to learn enough of your methods to make it through to the finish line. You are truly a hero and deserve so much of the credit for Cody's recovery.

Michael Warren: You are brilliant! Once you saw the evidence, you made deeper connections that have allowed you to help so many others. My prayer is that other medical professionals will follow suit.

Cindy Blom: You walked alongside me as I moved from sickness to health in more ways than I can count. Your willingness to learn about this and couple it with what you already knew gives me hope that others can and will do the same. Your son Erik's sacrifice was the driving factor to begin my work on the second book, *What's Wrong with Me: I'm an Addict*. Thank you for your time, intervention, and most of all, your unconditional love. Without you, there would be no book deal and no nutraceuticals. On behalf of those we may be able to reach with the second book, thank you.

Dad: You're a rock. Your stable influence on my life taught me to never give up, to think logically, and to trust but verify. Sitting down at night and working with me on Algebra II until we arrived at the correct answer for all the problems taught me to not stop until things made sense. You were my example for hard work, loyalty, dedication, and perseverance. Your unwavering support regardless of the situation gave me one thing that stayed the same through it all. And now, your work teaching children in detention centers because of what happened to Cody demonstrates your heart for those who need support. Thank you for being who you are.

Mom: Your life has been full of so many hardships, but you pushed through and never stopped searching for ways to get better. It was a beautiful thing to watch. I learned from you to not stop trying even when there were so many ups and downs. Your kindness and acceptance of others, no matter what was wrong with them, have always been so inspirational. Thank you for your sacrifices and for following what you believe with all your heart, mind, and strength. I learned how to do the same from you. You stood with me during all of the hell I went through with Judge Guffee. Thank you. You were right about Cody needing brain rehabilitation (as do countless others in our society).

Grandma Jinny: You are gone now, but I'll never forget you telling me all the time, "This too shall pass." I held onto that truth for dear life and prayed that you were right, which you were. Teaching me that an education was the most valuable thing I could do for myself and that independence was mandatory ended up saving our lives. Thank you.

To my children: I am so grateful that God trusted me enough to allow your precious souls into my life. Kelsey, Michelle, Adam, and Cody... I could not be prouder! I am so sorry this had to be our journey, but I am also so grateful that it was with the four of you. I look forward to the rest of our lives together and cannot wait to see what God has in store for your future. Today, each moment I have with you guys is my brightest moment.

John, the father of my children: Times were hard, and you did the best you could. Thank you for loving the children so much through it all.

Steven Harris: Your suffering was unimaginable, but your heart was so wonderful. You are in a better place now. No more suffering. We all loved you so much. I would give anything to go back in time and to have figured this out sooner for your sake. You loved life so much.

Andi Durkin: You didn't know me from Adam other than a Facebook post and agreed, sight unseen, to edit my manuscript. You had no idea who I was or even if the treatment would eventually work. Yet you spent countless hours helping me until the manuscript was accepted by a publisher! Without your guidance, I would not have known what to do with the thousand pages of gibberish I had typed up. You told me the story was in the last 250 pages. I could not believe it, the hardest part of the story. But you gently nudged me to document each doctor's visit, pull labs, and put together Cody's story with scientific and chronological accuracy. Thank you. Now we can help others. Your angels must have told you to do it because I was a wreck!

Dee Dee: Thank you for believing in me enough to do the job even in my unstable circumstances. And thank you for putting everything into making La Bella e Famosa of Green Hills perfect. With the right treatment, Cody was able to manage while you and I spent long days and nights opening the most fabulous spa Nashville has to offer.

Brittny Reid: You lived through it as a teenager and suffered greatly because of the effects of this on your young adult life. God brought you back to me for such a time and purpose as this. Your work ethic, drive, and commitment to the spa and this mission kept me going during the year of rebuilding, and while finishing the book. Your relentless pursuit of the truth brought you to your answers and you will help so many because of your story. Now, you can truly recover. You are a true example of the student becoming the teacher.

Kaaren Mayfield: Thank you for teaching me the principles which guided me throughout the darkest of times. The countless hours you invested paid off tremendously.

To all of the clients who patiently listened to me rattle on about things for years on end. Through your support and your ideas, I was able to get to the right answer.

Glynn Dilbeck: I was so broken by the time we finally found you. I had no idea how to manage the trauma Cody had endured and just barely was starting to get a handle on the PANDAS diagnosis. You have been patient, kind, and so valuable in terms of your competence and willingness. And you're an expert witness to top it all off. Thank you for your guidance and unwavering support of Cody.

Karen Anderson: Out of nowhere, you came into my life and made it possible for this story to reach the masses. An expert in your field, you were kind yet honest. So, I listened to you. You patiently waded through book dives and told me to keep going when I wanted to quit. Ten years to live it and another three to finish the book, but you left no option other than the finish line. And now, we are crossing it together. Morgan James Publishers was the perfect fit for me. Thank you for being a part of an agency focused on excellence and integrity.

Adéle Booysen: Your combination of empathy and strength is unparalleled. You walked me through the emotional decisions of editing this story, evidence of the devotion you have to your clients. Night and day, we worked for hundreds of hours to get this book to the place it is today. There is no way I could have done it without you. You are one of the most focused and committed professionals I have worked with throughout my career. Thank you for the encouragement I needed to finish my book.

ABOUT ELIZABETH HARRIS

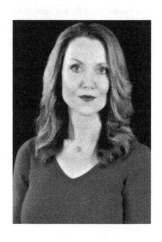

Elizabeth Harris waged a hard-fought battle to get to the root of her family's medical issues, especially the strange disease that hijacked her first-born son's life. Using her science education background and her experience as a successful entrepreneur, Elizabeth exposes the mysterious bacteria that is not only behind her son's disease but is also a key contributor to a myriad of maladies in America. Through What's Wrong Wellness, this mother of four spends much of her time educating medical professionals and other parents on her discoveries. In addition to thousands of hours of her own personal research, Elizabeth is expanding her knowledge by pursuing formal education in this field. At the time of publication, she was working toward earning a Master's in Molecular Medicine. She has learned that even today, although mycoplasma is recognized as being on rise, it is still recommended that children who are infected with mycoplasma and have liver involvement should be "followed conservatively to avoid unnecessary diagnostic procedures in the future." She resides in Franklin, Tennessee, where she owns a high-end wellness and medi-spa, and she continues to work toward a solution on behalf of the children.

A free ebook edition is available with the purchase of this book.

To claim your free ebook edition:

1. Visit MorganJamesBOGO.com
2. Sign your name CLEARLY in the space
3. Complete the form and submit a photo of the entire copyright page
4. You or your friend can download the ebook to your preferred device

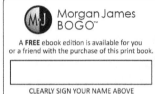

A **FREE** ebook edition is available for you or a friend with the purchase of this print book.

CLEARLY SIGN YOUR NAME ABOVE

Instructions to claim your free ebook edition:
1. Visit MorganJamesBOGO.com
2. Sign your name CLEARLY in the space above
3. Complete the form and submit a photo of this entire page
4. You or your friend can download the ebook to your preferred device

Print & Digital Together Forever.

Snap a photo

Free ebook

Read anywhere

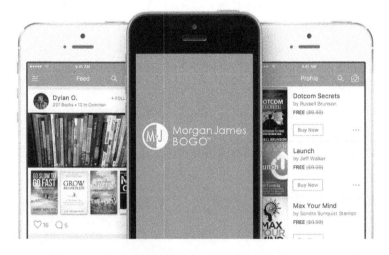

Printed in the USA
CPSIA information can be obtained
at www.ICGtesting.com
JSHW022320140824
68134JS00019B/1209

9 781631 954979